THE NURSE PRACTITIONERS' GUIDE TO AUTOIMMUNE MEDICINE

THE
NURSE
PRACTITIONERS'
GUIDE

TO AUTOIMMUNE MEDICINE

Reversing and Preventing
All Autoimmunity

DAVID BILSTROM, M.D.

The Nurse Practitioners' Guide to Autoimmune Medicine
Reversing and Preventing All Autoimmunity

ISBN: 978-1-7357922-1-7 (Hardcover)
ISBN: 978-1-7357922-0-0 (Paperback)

For permission requests or to get in touch with the author, please visit *www.DrDavidBilstrom.com*

Cover Design by: Nikyta Guleria

This book is dedicated to Jody, Dylan, and Tierney.

"How wonderful life is when you're in the world."

—ELTON JOHN

Autoimmune Medicine

"Got a revolution. Got to revolution."

—JEFFERSON AIRPLANE

NPSLEAD33

This is your special code to access additional information that supplements the book whenever you see a reference to *www.DrDavidBilstrom.com/npadguide*.

"This book is wonderful for anyone wanting to learn more about autoimmune disease and what to do about it. It is a great tool for both clinicians that want to improve outcomes in their AD patients as well as for individuals with AD that want to learn how to be advocates of their own health. Dr. Bilstrom's vision of preventing and reversing autoimmune disease will be exponentially more attainable as this book gets onto the shelves of as many healthcare offices & homes as possible!"

— Christina Stapke, RDN, CD
Contributor to Integrative & Functional Medical Nutrition Therapy: Principles & Practices (2020)

TABLE OF CONTENTS

ABOUT THE AUTHOR

David Bilstrom, M.D. is a fellow of the American Academy of Integrative Medicine and American Academy of Medical Acupuncture as well as an advanced fellow in anti-aging, regenerative, and functional medicine. Dr. David Bilstrom is quadruple board certified in Anti-aging and Regenerative Medicine, Integrative Medicine, Physical Medicine & Rehabilitation, and Medical Acupuncture.

Dr. Bilstrom is the Director of the International Autoimmune Institute and the Bingham Memorial Center for Functional Medicine—the first medical center in the country associated with a teaching hospital to treat all types of autoimmune diseases.

Dr. Bilstrom is devoted to educating medical professionals on the effectiveness of treating and preventing autoimmune disease rather than just symptom controlled medications that cause additional illness. Improving the patient's experience and quality of life.

WHY WRITE A GUIDE ON REVERSING AND PREVENTING ALL AUTOIMMUNE DISEASE?

Whoever is happy will make others happy too.

—ANNE FRANK

THE SCOPE OF THE PROBLEM

Autoimmune disease (AD) affects millions of people worldwide. It's a leading cause of death among female children and women 65 years and younger.[1] One hundred billion dollars is spent every year in the United States for AD-related care, while fifty billion is spent on all cancer care.[1] However, the NIH spends only $591 million on AD research compared to the $6.1 billion spent every year on cancer research.[1] In fact, AD is the most popular health topic requested by calls made to the National Women's Health Information Center. This makes sense because 80% of people who get an autoimmune disease are women.

TYPICAL TREATMENT OPTIONS AND THEIR PROBLEMS

Often, when someone is diagnosed with AD, they are offered medications that push the immune system "down" in an attempt to suppress the overactive part of immune system dysregulation. So, it makes sense when the person is advised that these medications will increase their chance of getting cancer or an infection that could lead to death.

It is important to understand that the medications often used in patients with ADs do not correct the problem. They only put a temporary band-aid on the symptoms. If an individual feels bad enough they can't come close to getting through their day, a band-aid may be a good place to start. However, without fixing the reasons why they developed the AD in the first place, the individual will likely become sicker and risk getting new ADs that develop into new chronic diseases.

If we spent more time addressing the underlying mechanism of the disease and not just the symptoms, people would be less prone to illness. In our current world, this is not often the case. Using typical medicines can be okay. It is best to use them to buy time; to do the appropriate testing, address what is found, and reverse the underlying processes and current symptoms so the patient starts feeling better, and then wean down and off the medications. Once off the meds, they will no longer have to worry about the potential side effects, which sometimes include death.

When a person presents with an AD, we are in a unique position to stop the attack and allow the symptoms to reverse and the body to heal. AD often begins with a long history of events that negatively impact the immune system; sometimes beginning years or decades before a diagnosis.

A STORY: GLENN FREY OF THE EAGLES

One of the reasons I am so passionate about AD is the story of Glenn Frey of the American rock band The Eagles. What occurred with Glenn should never happen to anyone but is typical for many people with ADs. Here is Glenn Frey, diagnosed with Rheumatoid Arthritis (RA), an AD that eventually destroys the affected joints. He is prescribed the typical medicines for ADs. However, they don't fix the underlying reasons why the immune system attacks specific body parts in the first place. Further, because the underlying issues were not addressed, the problem kept getting worse. Glenn died in January 2016. By all accounts after his death, he had not felt well for years but had tried hard not to show his suffering. These were accounts from two of his best friends; Bob Seger and Jackson Brown.

Did Glenn Frey die from RA? No. He died of acute ulcerative colitis and pneumonia that no amount of antibiotics could clear because his immune system was so suppressed.[2] He died from the autoimmune disease process just getting worse until he developed a subsequent AD; a new or "acute" AD that attacked his intestines, his gut. Since he was already at an increased risk of infection due to the underlying immune system dysregulation, antibiotics were useless. Further, the immunosuppressant medication he was on increases the risk of antibiotic-resistant infections. This scenario is happening around the world. There are even thousands of documented occurrences of these types of medications causing a new AD to develop as a side effect.[3,4]

BILSTROM'S NUCLEARITIS

An ounce of prevention is worth a pound of cure.

—Benjamin Franklin

Let's discuss an AD that didn't have a name until 2018 and thus no treatment would begin until the person's situation was so dire, their quality of life so poor, that they had almost no choice but to start the typical medicines with the typical profound downsides.

Bilstrom's Nuclearitis. Noun. A chronic autoimmune disease characterized by the production of antibodies which mistakenly attack proteins in the nucleus of cells within the human body including structures such as DNA. First described by American physiatrist, functional medicine and integrative medicine physician David Bilstrom in 2018.

Autoimmune diseases don't start as autoimmune diseases. They start years or decades earlier as very small adverse biochemical alterations that the body's self-correcting mechanisms are not able to fix. It can take 10-20 years before the very first symptoms actually start and then much longer before the actual diagnosis of an AD occurs.

In order to prevent autoimmune disease, it's important to recognize the immune system dysregulation long before someone is bad enough to actually be diagnosed with an AD. One example of a reasonable initial intervention would be the use of biologics. Hopefully, as we educate the world about reversing and preventing ADs, you will recognize more and more young people with early signs of immune system disruption. Early signs in young children include Eczema, allergies, asthma, recurrent infections of any kind, and even cancer may be the first sign of the immune system going down the road towards AD. Knowledge is essential to not only reverse the current symptoms but prevent the development of an AD long term.

Bilstrom's Nuclearitis is an AD that occurs when a person tests positive for antinuclear antibodies, a positive ANA, without other antibodies being produced that would signify a definitive diagnosis of lupus or rheumatoid arthritis, for example. Now that we have a named disease to go with a positive ANA, treatment can be initiated potentially years earlier, rather than waiting until additional body parts start being attacked and the patient's functional status and quality of life are so compromised that medications like immunosuppressants, NSAIDs, and opioids must be the first line of treatment.

Having a proper name for the disease which occurs when the ANA is positive helps to initiate proper treatment earlier than the typical timeline. Particularly when it is the first antibody to be produced, the autoimmune process can hopefully be reversed before the immune system starts to attack new body structures. If a person is producing thyroid antibodies along with the positive ANA, the TPO and thyroglobulin antibodies can be a nice way to track how well the immune system dysregulation process is being reversed, right along with how well the person is feeling. The goal here is for the thyroid antibody numbers to go down to zero and the ANA to turn negative.

Bilstrom's Nuclearitis occurs so often. Studies have found that 16% of US women have a positive ANA. This is almost 30 million women. Is Bilstrom's Nuclearitis the most common autoimmune disease of all? Not even the rich and famous are immune. What famous person (who is wonderful in so many ways, including her work with at-risk youth and adults) has an aunt with lupus? Has had to cancel tour dates because of health issues? Has been identified as having a positive ANA "but no autoimmune disease or lupus like her aunt?" Has been told that "fibromyalgia" is the source of her health issues? Lady Gaga.

This newly identified disease is an example of how far reaching your impact can be when you fully understand immune system dysregulation.

MASTERS DO THE BASICS WELL

Your time is limited, so don't waste it living someone else's life. Don't be trapped by dogma- living with the results of other people's thinking.

—Steve Jobs

WHY A BOOK ON THE BASICS IS NEEDED

This book was written with the simple goal of changing the way all autoimmune diseases are treated and prevented worldwide. For this to happen, there needs to be an expert on how to do this in every community. To be experts, people first need to realize that the reversal and prevention of all autoimmune diseases is possible. Hence, there needs to be at least one patient-focused, holistically-minded medical professional who has the desire to change the world starting with their community. Nurse practitioners seem to be the logical choice, given their training, mindset, and oftentimes central role in the health of their families.

This journey is for you if you are a medical professional who recognizes we are not doing what's best for our patients (and the world) when we wait for these diseases to become manifested in families, generation after generation, and only offer medication that puts a temporary bandage on one particular body part. You are well-suited to transform generations of lives providing the compassionate care that brought you into medicine in the first place.

If you've had basic training in traditional allopathic medicine, you can easily be trained in the basics to make a profound, multi-organ system, impact on every patient. Also, thousands of medical professionals every year make an effort to acquire this "new knowledge" to transform the way they practice medicine. Oftentimes, they may be spurred on by significant medical issues; one that is not responding . to the interventions considered traditional allopathic medicine. They may have already searched for some nontraditional treatments and the person(s) of concern are not improving.

Thus, they tell themselves,

> "If I can't find someone who can fix my daughter's problem (or son, or spouse, or parent, etc…), I will figure out how to do it myself."

They then attend a functional or integrative medicine conference. They can't believe how:

- great the scientific information is,
- much is known about reversing and preventing chronic disease,
- they didn't know this information even existed,
- impactful this could be on their loved ones and patients,
- they went through their entire medical training and were never taught this.

They return to their medical practice on Monday morning with a renewed spirit and excitement they may not have felt for years. Motivated to use the newly acquired knowledge to change the world but they get stuck! They have all this new wisdom but don't know how to start. They might need to put off making changes until they have more time. Then seldom get the time. After a couple of months, it's too late.

When I attend these conferences, I sit next to people from all over the world and I ask, "How long have you been coming to these conferences?" They often reply by saying something like, "Oh, I'm a member of the Academy and I have been coming here for 10 years." Then I inquire, "What kind of functional/integrative medicine practice do you do?" Now, before I tell you what their response always is, let me add that I started this journey almost 3 decades ago. When it comes to the medicine I practice nowadays, I had to dive right in, full tilt, due to my child's health issues. All other options had been exhausted. So for me, it was easy; I learned it, I did it.

The response I always hear,

> "Oh, I'm still just a traditional _____ (insert the name of any medical specialty here). I use some of it at home though. With my family. We take supplements. It's so fascinating. I love to learn about it. I just have never figured out how to do it at work."

WOW!

I concluded that learning this detailed science is fascinating— (enough to keep practitioners coming back year after year) but how to do the work is elusive. You have to teach yourself the day-in-day-out, nuts and bolts, of how to actually care for the patient.

All the esoteric knowledge, no matter how wonderful, doesn't tell you:

- What form a patient should fill out?
- How to scan all the information on the history form to quickly discern what is wrong?
- What type of tests to order (and the expected results of these tests) even before meeting the patient?

- What specific tests need to be run, and why?
- What blood work needs to be written for and run at the hospital or local lab?
- How to analyze and interpret the lab data that comes back and what instructions should the patient get?
- When to retest and how to make the appropriate changes in management based on this new data?
- How to make sure that the patient stays healthy for the next 50 years?

Perhaps the decision-making processes described above sounds familiar. It should. This is what we as medical practitioners do every day. It should be easy. And it is. We can do this with our eyes closed. The problem is, the medical practitioner doesn't know the basics of reversing and preventing autoimmune disease and all disease as a whole. This is not what we're taught in school. A medical professional may have learned a lot of great scientific information from their years of going to functional and integrative medical conferences but they don't know the basics. This is why, the organization that I love so much (and has done so much to help me get to this point), has over 15,000 members worldwide but the person sitting next to me keeps repeating "I still just practice "regular" medicine."

Maybe we are doing this backward? A good friend of mine, a physical therapist, once said, "masters do the basics well." When you know the basics of how to reverse and prevent all ADs you should be able to do at least 60-70-80% of what needs to be done for patients and families! After watching patients get much better than they ever imagined (remember, most AD patients see 4-5 healthcare providers over 3-5 years before even getting the diagnosis explaining their chronic symptoms let alone finding someone to reverse the process), then, you can always learn more and fine-tune your ability to practice this kind of medicine. Remember, masters do the basics well.

This book provides the knowledge to do just that. I've seen it happen already with my physician extender. Why not everyone else? Why not with at least one nurse practitioner in every community worldwide? Learn the nuts and bolts. Become an expert in your community. Help people that no one else can help. Gain the knowledge to help your family reverse any chronic health issues and stay healthy for the next 80 years. Okay, maybe just 25-30 years if they are already 70.

HOW TO USE
THIS BOOK

The question isn't who is going to let me;
it's who is going to stop me.

—Ayn Rand

Now you know:

1. Autoimmune disease is a major problem.
2. The way ADs are treated is a big problem.
3. Masters do the basics well.

If you can master the basics, you will become a master: the local expert in reversing and preventing all autoimmunity in your community, and beyond. Our International Autoimmune Institute is an excellent example. We are a medical tourism destination because people with ADs are willing to come from all over the world for the care they cannot get close to home.

To master the basics and translate this into clinical patient care, become familiar with the first five chapters for a good foundation:

1. Why Write a Guide on Reversing and Preventing Autoimmune Disease?
2. Masters Do the Basics Well... Why a Book on the Basics is Needed
3. How to Use This Book

4. Overview of Immune System Regulation
5. Causes of Autoimmune Disease

This information is great to share with patients. It can be life-changing. Often they have seen many doctors and endured many years of suffering by the time they find you. This will also be the knowledge needed to explain why they got their AD, how to reverse it, and prevent getting new ones. There is no better way to learn something than to teach it to others. Teaching the basics to all your patients over and over again will be vital in becoming the "expert" in this type of medicine. A master of the basics.

Because what causes ADs is a big driver of all diseases, it's common to reverse all health issues even if not related to an autoimmune process. By doing it this way, there is due diligence in preventing future disease as well. The very best in preventative medicine.

Once the information in these five chapters is perused, the "Diagnostic Testing" chapter will make sense. This chapter contains information such as what blood tests to order through your local hospital or lab and what tests require in-office testing kits for patients at the time of their visit.

Get familiar with these tests and the information they supply. It will then be easy to explain to the patient what testing is needed and why. You can say,.

- We need to do a blood test to look at a few vitamins and minerals, not a lot, but just a few.
- We need to look really closely at your hormones.
- We will look for the chronic infections that contribute to these types of ADs.
- We will test for celiac disease even if you've had it looked at before.

- We need to do a saliva cortisol test to get a good look at what is going on with the 'stress' hormone cortisol. Cortisol always gets thrown off in these situations. Saliva testing is more accurate than blood testing and it was the original cortisol test.
- We need to do a stool test to find out exactly what is going on in the gut. The gut is a central mechanism for AD and all diseases.
- We also need to do a food sensitivity test. This is a finger prick test that will tell us what foods are bothering you, creating issues, but doing it in a "sneaky" way. They may not bother you right away after you eat them but they create inflammation, days or weeks later. Thus you may find yourself saying, "Holy cow, I'm not feeling nearly as well as I should be. I'm not 100 years old. I need to figure out what is going on! I want to feel better and not keep getting worse and worse." With this test, we can figure out what foods make you sick without you knowing it. We will have you avoid them, at least temporarily, and this will open up the window of opportunity to fix everything.
- Eventually, we will do a urine test to check for environmental toxins. This test looks for lead, mercury, arsenic, cadmium, aluminum, even uranium. Environmental toxins are one reason why researchers believe so many more people have ADs now compared to a few years ago.

The "Treatment Options to Consider at the Time of the First Visit" chapter, has powerful options to potentially start right away, even before the patient returns for their follow-up to review the lab results. At first, consider writing down a summary of these options to have available in the exam room while going over the patient's "plan of action" at the end of the first visit. Eventually, you will know this information backward and forward.

The "Test Interpretation" chapter: In the beginning, go over the results sheets before entering the exam room and going over the lab results with the patient, and if present, their family members. Having chronic AD(s) affects the entire family and family dynamics. Everyone has a vested interest in the person with AD finding the correct medical practitioner and getting well.

Write down on the blood work results sheets the optimal ranges for the labs to be discussed with the patient. Use an "up" or "down" arrow to indicate if the patient's result is either too high or too low compared to the optimal range. Make notes and comments on the results sheets from all the advanced testing ordered. This includes the testing kits that needed to be mailed in by the patient. When entering the patient's room, you will have everything needed to go over the labs "with a fine-tooth comb". Over time, this becomes simple. Pre-visit preparation will be unnecessary.

The blood work optimal ranges will be the slowest ones to memorize but in the process of becoming a master, it will happen. In the beginning, keep the optimal ranges for all the blood tests on one page, in front of you, as you review the patient's results. These are available for download at www.DrDavidBilstrom.com/npadguide.

This next part is critical! Once you have reviewed all this with your patient, look them in the eye, pause for a moment, and then say something like...

> "Wow, isn't it great to finally know exactly why you have been feeling so bad for so long? No wonder you're feeling so bad. Who's going to feel great with all this going on?"

The patient will likely feel overwhelmed. But also, relieved to know that they have <u>finally</u> found someone who can tell them why they have felt so bad for so long. They might have spent years going from one medical person to another and never got the answers. Such as, "Why did I get this?" "Can I make this go away?" And if so, "How can I make this go away?"

Many times, people start to cry at this point. They may have already cried during their first visit as they realize they have finally found the person who knows why they got this AD and knows how to make it go away. During this second visit though, you have now validated all the symptoms they've had for many years.

This is extremely important. They may say, "You mean this is not just all in my head? I'm not going crazy?" For most medical practitioners, it is so confusing when a patient has problems in every organ system all at the same time. Now, this next part is terrible but true. In this situation, many women have been told, "You're just depressed." How terrible! No medical practitioner would ever say this to a man. If they did they probably would get punched. Yet, women hear this all the time. So when you have just validated that they are not "just crazy" tears may come. The healing has already started.

You can tell the patient:

> "It is so confusing for most medical people when every organ system is off at the same time. But for medical people like "us," it makes it easy. The only way everything can be off at the same time is because important central mechanisms have been thrown off. The central mechanisms that create all disease, not just AD. The vitamins and minerals, hormones, stress and the stress hormone cortisol, chronic infections, toxins, food sensitivities, and the gut. By identifying exactly what is going on with the advanced testing we've done, we should be in a good position to fix everything at the same time. Because they are all connected."

This is life-changing for the patient and their family.

In the next three chapters: "Treatment Options Based on Lab Data," "When and What to Retest," and "When to Simplify and What to Use Long Term," first get familiar with the information in general but don't try to memorize it right away.

Also, get familiar with how these chapters are set up. Initially, keep this book in the room with the patient while making recommendations based on the lab test results. It will help to have the handout on optimal ranges in the blood work, and this book for easy to access information regarding these three chapters. Patients will not mind if this information is with you while making treatment decisions. They are so thrilled to have found the person they have been looking for all these years; and that there is specific scientific data to identify why they got AD and how to reverse the process.

The "Long Term Follow-Up" chapter is self-explanatory. Get familiar with the information as far as understanding what a patient's needs will be long term. It will complete the "picture" you will "paint" for the patient while going over the labs in their initial follow-up visit. The visit includes making recommendations for a variety of supplements/medications and essential lifestyle changes. Oftentimes, the initial supplement/medication regimen will include quite a few items.

I tell patients,

> "It always takes more to get good than to stay good."

> "Once you are 70-80-90% better overall, and your repeat labs look much better, we will be in a position to start weaning down and coming off most of these supplements and medications. This will most likely include the medications that suppress your immune system and have many long-term side effects."

By this time you will have been able to get them off all the other meds with significant side effects and negative impacts on the gut and the body such as NSAIDs, acid-blocking medicines, metformin, and BCPs to name a few.

You can finish by telling the patient,

> "If all goes well, eventually you may only need daily vitamin D, the low dose Naltrexone, and once a week a probiotic. Maybe a multivitamin. Maybe some fish oil. We will see."

In the chapter titled "Providing Supplement Access for Your Patients," you will learn why it is crucial to provide patients with high-quality supplements. These are often called "nutraceuticals." A person will never turn around these stubborn, chronic ADs with over-the-counter (OTC) supplements they find in their local chain stores. You will find fascinating the information regarding what a person is getting in their capsules when not using "nutraceuticals." A patient needs products that contain what the label lists and nothing else. There should be enough of the active ingredient to turn the chronic disease around. We will review both short-term and long-term options, including, why having them available for patients through your office may be ideal. You will also get information about using compounding pharmacies and how to get the testing kits patients will need.

In the "Addendum" section, you will learn how to enhance your knowledge with the information from an upcoming book. This new book will provide much more detailed information on all the subjects discussed in this guide. This will include more about cortisol and thyroid conversion, for example. First steps first. Master the basics and become an expert by teaching others. Patients in your community are in dire need of it. Thank you for joining with me to create a revolution to change the way autoimmune diseases are treated and prevented worldwide.

OVERVIEW OF IMMUNE SYSTEM DYSREGULATION

*How wonderful it is that nobody need wait a single
moment before starting to improve the world.*

—Anne Frank.

THE SIMULTANEOUS UPREGULATED AND DOWNREGULATED IMMUNE SYSTEM

What needs to happen to get a person's immune system so disrupted that their body attacks itself and they develop an AD? At this point, the body is self-destructing. As with most things in our world, there is a sweet spot to achieving balance and harmony. We should not be too high or too low. It's like driving on a highway—the speed limit tends to reflect that sweet spot. Driving too fast or too slow is dangerous. The sweet spot right in the middle helps traffic flow effectively. When a person loses the sweet spot in their immune system, they will move away from it both up and down at the same time.

Upregulated immune system issues include allergies, asthma, eczema, and all the ADs. The down-regulated immune system can lead to colds, cases of the flu, infections, recurrent infections, and cancer.[4] As time goes by, it is easy to develop new immune system issues on top of old ones. It is easy to deduce that when a person develops one AD, they are more likely to get a second, third, fourth, or even fifth.[5]

When a person is diagnosed with AD, they are offered medications that suppress the overactive portion of the immune system disruption. However, only addressing the overactive immune system issues can create even worse down-regulated immune system issues, thus, leading to an increased risk of cancer and infections.

If a person's immune system dysregulation caused an AD but also an increased risk of infections and cancer, and now the recommended medication causes an even greater risk of these illnesses, something is not right. The immune system agrees. It doesn't want suppression. It wants to be rebalanced (also known as immune system modulation) reestablishing the immune system set point.

AUTOIMMUNE DISEASE IS ONE BIG DISEASE

It is vital to understand that there are not hundreds of autoimmune diseases requiring hundreds of treatment strategies. In reality, there is only one big disease that can affect a system and/or any aspect of the human body. From entire organs—such as Hashimoto's to individual enzymes, like osteoporosis, and even membrane channels, including voltage-gated potassium channels (VGKCs) in neurologic disease. Thus, it becomes easy to get a "second" autoimmune disease after the "first." And then a "third," "fourth," and "fifth".

One disease that goes after the most fragile spot in the body first. Then, it will attack the second weakest spot, then the third, etc. Some have suggested this one big disease could be called "Poly-autoimmunity." However, more recently, this has just been a term used to describe a person with more than one AD at the same time. This term refers to anyone who is identified as having an AD, but no one bothered to determine why they got it and reverse the process before getting a second AD. Instead, their AD was given the time for the immune system to start attacking new body parts.

CAUSES
OF AUTOIMMUNE DISEASE

Life is either a daring adventure or nothing at all.

—Helen Keller

So, what causes the immune system to lose that sweet spot right in the middle and move away both up and down at the same time? Vitamin deficiencies, hormone imbalances and deficiencies, toxic stress and cortisol issues, environmental toxins, chronic infections, and gut imbalances, just to name a few.[6,7,8,9,10,11] See figures 1 and 2.

Allergies, Asthma, Autoimmune Disease

Immune system set point

Colds, Flus, Infections,
Recurrent Infections & Cancer

Figure 1

Causes for Loss of Immune System Set Point

■ Vitamin and mineral defincies

■ Hormone imbalance or deficiencies

■ Toxicity including toxic stress

■ Infections

■ The gut

Figure 2

The gut is the central mechanism because once it is disrupted enough it will cause all the other issues or cause them to get worse. When the gut is a problem, it will be difficult to digest and absorb the nutrients from food. When the gut is off, it will negatively impact hormone balance. The gut in fact makes some vital hormones, such as melatonin. Low levels of melatonin have been linked to chronic diseases, such as Alzheimer's, stroke, heart attacks, cancer, and many pain problems including fibromyalgia, pelvic pain, and headaches such as migraines, cluster headaches, and tension headaches.[12,13] When the gut is off, toxins will not efficiently be cleared from the body. This includes internally generated toxins that every cell in the body makes as toxic byproducts of metabolism. As well as the many environmental toxins that found their way into our bodies. When the gut is off, it has a direct negative impact on the immune system as 80% of the immune system surrounds the gut.[14] Once that is disrupted, troublesome microorganisms will get into the body and help drive AD.

Knowing what triggers immune system dysregulation will make it easy to decide what tests to run to treat each individual. Many, if not all symptoms, are often driven by the same predicament that caused AD in the first place.

Initial Blood Work Men Only - In addition to
Basic Blood Work for Both Sexes

TT (Total Testosterone)
Free T (Free Testosterone)
DHT (Dihydrotestosterone)
Estradiol
Estrone

Dr. David
Bilstrom

Nutrients. We want to examine certain vitamin and mineral levels during our investigation. Tests exist that can calculate the levels of up to 100 essential nutrients. However, it is reasonable to start small with a few key tests often found in a hospital or traditional lab. As gut health improves and gets better at digesting and absorbing nutrients, the body will repair many nutritional deficiencies even if they were not part of the original testing. The body is smarter than we realize. The neat thing is that we don't have to go after every problem. We just need to pursue and attack the "biggest fish to fry" and the body will sort the rest out by itself.

Hormones. When it comes to hormones, it is essential to look at the big picture. The patient needs a thorough overview of many hormones, and they need to be done at the same time. Think of hormones as a big symphony orchestra. All the players are critical on an individual level. However, what might be more important is how they collaborate. It takes just one player to falter, and they will disrupt the entire orchestra. The same applies to hormones. Each hormone is crucial. What might be more essential is how they work together. All it takes is one hormone to be off, and it will throw off all the others. Thus, start wondering about all the other hormones when one is off.

If the symphony is off, it's essential to fix it. One cannot just look at the woodwind section to figure out what is going on. Review the entire orchestra to determine what is throwing it off. Within this symphony of hormones is a tight triad: Cortisol, thyroid, and insulin/blood sugar (see Figure 4). Just like any triangle in space, changing one angle will change the other two. When the thyroid gets thrown off, insulin and blood sugar are also usually thrown off in AD patients.[8,9] When cortisol and thyroid are off; it almost always creates problems with blood sugar control.[8,9] Thus, insulin resistance will often fix itself once you fix the big picture.

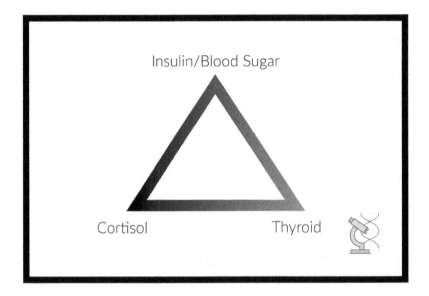

Figure 4

Chronic Infections. Chronic infections can, and often do, lead to AD. As previously mentioned, with a dysfunctional immune system, we get down-regulated issues simultaneous with the up-regulated issues. Remember that down-regulated immune system issues include colds, cases of the flu, chronic viral and bacterial infections, recurrent infections, and cancer. As time has gone on, more literature has been published about how chronic infections can drive AD, however, research is still developing. For example, a 2015 article discussed a new microorganism found in the throat that appears to drive the development of schizophrenia.[15] The oropharynx microbiome difference between patients and controls could be used to predict the future of disease diagnosis.[15]

It is not surprising that chronic infections often lead to AD, given what we already know about chronic infections in the gut driving disease. The gut is such a central mechanism in all diseases (not just within the gut), and it can drive many different body and brain issues. In many ways, the "gut" is just one big long tube—starting at the nose/mouth all the way to the rectum. Chronic infections in the stomach, like H. Pylori, or in the small intestines, like Small Bowel Bacterial Overgrowth (SIBO), drive other diseases. Microorganisms in the mouth can cause gingivitis but also cardiovascular disease.[16] Chronic fungal infections in the sinuses can cause headaches and chronic sinusitis,[17] with subsequent supra-infections involving bacteria. However, the use of antibiotics doesn't eliminate the fungal infection and the person continues to suffer from chronic sinusitis. Then, they may get recurring bacterial infections. In due course, they are faced with surgery, but because the underlying fungal infection is still present, they will continue getting sinus symptoms. They may undergo multiple sinus surgeries.

Celiac Disease. Without exception, testing for celiac disease (CD) needs to be done in every patient unless they have already been diagnosed with CD. Also, be mindful of the increased risk of CD when a person already has one or more of the following AD: type 1 diabetes (T1DM), rheumatoid arthritis, Hashimoto's thyroiditis, autoimmune hepatitis, and Sjogren's. When someone has an untreated CD, all sorts of problems can occur: anemia, osteoporosis, infertility and miscarriage, epilepsy, short stature, heart disease, and intestinal cancers, just to name a few.[18] Painful conditions can develop, such as headaches and migraines, joint pain/arthritis, peripheral neuropathy, and bone fractures. The untreated CD can also cause agonizing ADs such as TIDM, multiple sclerosis (MS), and dermatitis herpetiformis.[18,19] Only 20% of people suffering from CD are ever diagnosed. Why? Only 20% of people have significant GI symptoms and experience what is called a "classic CD." Meanwhile, 80% of individuals with CD have minimal or no GI symptoms, or an "atypical CD."[19,20]

Anticipating Future Disease. All the testing will not only tell us why they developed AD and chronic diseases in general but will also tell us where they are going. If they are moving toward diabetes, cardiovascular disease, Alzheimer's, osteoporosis, rheumatoid arthritis, Lupus, or celiac disease, for example, we want to be aware so we can turn that ship around. TPO (thyroperoxidase) and thyroglobulin antibodies need to be checked on everyone with an AD (or just the TPO ABs in someone without a known AD) to see if they have developed an autoimmune process involving the thyroid. Whether it is an early autoimmune thyroid process or an already full-blown Hashimoto's thyroiditis.

SALIVA CORTISOL TESTING

One hormone that must be checked with saliva and not blood is cortisol. Saliva testing was the first technique developed to test for cortisol.[21] It is also the best way to examine intracellular levels of cortisol.[22] What occurs in our cells is more important than what is going on in the liquid part of our blood; the serum. Also keep in mind that the worst time to check a level of the "stress hormone" cortisol is right after stabbing the person with a sharp object, which is what a blood draw is. Spitting tends to be less stressful. To get an accurate reading of cortisol levels, they should be checked at 8 AM, noon, 5 PM, and 10 PM.[23] Saliva cortisol testing kits are available from several companies. We will discuss specific testing companies later in this book.

The Bilstrom Belly

Note: "The Bilstrom Belly." A fun physical exam finding that you will see (feel actually) quite often in people with bad cortisol disruption is the "Bilstrom Belly." I have never seen this described in the literature or heard mentioned in all my advanced training, but it's common in the office. Thus, I eventually had to give it a name. Cortisol has a large impact on blood flow. One of the ways that cortisol disruption has such a negative impact on gut function is its tendency to shunt blood flow away, thus depriving the gut of not only much-needed blood flow but also oxygen and nutrients. This lack of blood flow can make the abdomen cold to touch. The back of our hand is more temperature-sensitive than our palm. Hence, test during the physical examination. Have the patient adjust their clothing to expose the entire abdomen. Using the back of your hand, feel the temperature over different portions of the abdomen. Sometimes, you will find a subtle coldness over one portion of the abdomen compared to another. At other times a tremendous coldness over just one portion or the entire abdomen. It can be ice cold. It is so dramatic. The extreme cold can be felt before their abdomen is touched. When using a stethoscope to listen for bowel sounds (listen to the abdomen before touching it; as always) the cold might be radiating up to your hand. Both students rotating through my clinics and the patients themselves, have found this fascinating when I show them the "Bilstrom Belly." It is a great teaching tool to help people understand the tremendous impact that cortisol disruption has on gut function.

When I point out to patients their cold abdomen and tell them it has to do with cortisol issues, they sometimes will say,

"Oh my gosh! I have had this forever and no one could tell me why."

At other times, this will be the first time the person has noticed it. Either way, they will be even more excited to see the results of the saliva cortisol testing after experiencing the "Bilstrom Belly" physical exam.

DIGESTIVE STOOL ANALYSIS

The gut is an (if not THE) essential central mechanism driving AD and immune system dysregulation in general. As mentioned earlier, 80% of the immune system surrounds the gut, so it makes sense that gut dysfunction can affect the immune system. However, gut dysfunction can also lead to the development of other AD causes. We see more evidence every day that the gut is central to chronic disease.

When someone has diarrhea, constipation, gastroesophageal reflux disease (GERD), bloating, flatulence, foul-smelling stools, nausea, abdominal pain, undigested food in their stool, and bloody stools, it doesn't take a rocket scientist to figure out that a significant gut issue is transpiring. However, because the gut is such a central mechanism, a person may have no symptoms but the disrupted gut is creating all kinds of organ systems to be dysfunctional. This is why 8 out of 10 people with celiac disease don't even have gut symptoms. Despite having an AD attack on the small intestine, 80% of celiac patients have minimal or no gut symptoms.[19]

Food can't be digested and nutrients are not properly absorbed into the body. These nutrients are the basic building blocks the body uses to process, correct things, and be happy and healthy. The gut is called the "second brain" for a good reason. With the way current research is going, it is plausible the gut may be the "first brain." For now, let's continue to think of the gut as the "second brain."

The gut creates many items the brain needs to function, including the neurotransmitters serotonin and GABA.[24] For example, 90% of serotonin is made in the gut.[24] Serotonin is not entirely made by the gut for his good friend, the brain. The gut uses this neurotransmitter for purposes such as regulation of gut motility.

Serotonin is known for its effect on mood, but it also has a significant impact on the immune system, sleep, diabetes mellitus, autism spectrum disorder, Parkinson's, and Alzheimer's disease.[24] It's only logical that disrupted serotonin production would affect gut motility, mood, sleep, and the immune system all at once.

The gut is a vital organ for detoxification.[25] Every cell in our body makes toxic byproducts of metabolism. One internally generated toxin is so harmful that it must leave our bodies through breathing. While we need oxygen to survive, the toxic byproduct of oxygen metabolism is carbon dioxide. If carbon dioxide isn't removed from the body, it will kill us. Unfortunately, we live in a very toxic world swimming with lead, mercury, arsenic, pesticides, herbicides, plastics, and flame retardants, just to name a few. Our bodies have to clear them from our system. If we can't, they accumulate and create issues. Indeed, some toxins are excreted via urine, perspiration, or respirations, however, most are expelled through defecation. This includes internally generated and environmental toxins. If a person is not having at least one bowel movement per day, then various toxins and waste products are retained rather than eliminated as they should.

Clearing toxins from the body is essential. If the body is unable to clear old, toxic estrogens, it can lead to estrogen dominance. It isn't optimal for men either, but in women, the inability to clear old estrogen from the body is a significant driver of autoimmune disease. If the bowels are not functioning with a minimum of one daily bowel movement, then waste products and hormone metabolites are not eliminated as they should be. This is one explanation why 80% of individuals who get AD are women. Estrogen dominance is also a big reason why women get so many health issues that inform the knowledgeable medical practitioner that AD is approaching. Too much estrogen compared with progesterone is a big driver of excessive menstrual pain, heavy flows, premenstrual syndrome, PMDD, fibroids, endometriosis, ovarian cysts, and fibrocystic breast disease.[26] These health issues can begin to appear decades before the AD starts. This gives us plenty of time to fix the problem and prevent the AD from starting. By correcting these issues before a woman conceives, better gene expression is passed on; thus preventing AD and chronic disease in future generations. This is epigenetics. The scope of this book doesn't allow us to get into epigenetics at any depth. But suffice to say, epigenetics is captivating and we will cover it in our future work together. By the way, men need to optimize epigenetics before conception as well!

PROVOCATIVE HEAVY METAL TEST

There has been a significant increase in environmental toxins in our world, which has led to a significant increase in ADs.[27] In 1997, nine million people in the US were estimated to have an AD. Today, the number is closer to 50 million people with at least one AD, and almost 80% are women.[1,28,29] Rates are rising in Europe and other parts of the world. For example, Rheumatoid arthritis was unheard of in Japan for thousands of years, but now it is common.[30,31]

"Water-soluble toxins are not as big a problem as fat-soluble toxins."[32]

Water-soluble toxins are also easier to clear from the body. Fat-soluble toxins get stuck in our fat deposits and leach into our system, damaging the body and increasing the risk for chronic disease and disruption of the immune system. Did you know that our brains are 60% fat?[33] Because of this, they are super sensitive to fat-soluble toxins. Thus, the brain issues that we often see in people with AD are not just arising from the gut or hormones but also toxins. Common issues might include depression, anxiety, irritability, panic attacks, nightmares, memory and concentration issues, and much more.

Lead is a huge problem when it comes to chronic disease. A recent article suggested that perhaps 50% of all heart attacks in the US were due to lead.[34] Lead is so toxic to the cardiovascular system, even amounts we would not think were significant can have a negative impact.[35]

Proximally, 94% of lead sequesters in our bones and teeth.[36] Just having this amount of lead can cause some damage but something else happens at the time of menopause and andropause. The gradual (or fast as the case may be) loss of bone density allows the lead to flood into our system. Lead can disrupt all our organs, including the immune system. Can we just test for the lead in the bloodstream and confirm if it is an issue? No. Lead is fat-soluble, therefore, only trace amounts will be present in the water-soluble compartments, like blood serum, at any one time, even if there is plenty in our fat stores. Thus, blood tests for lead will underestimate how much is in the system. If even small amounts of lead are found in a blood test, the person can have a high toxic load in their body.

To pull the toxins from the fat stores into the urine to be tested, a provocative toxic heavy metal test needs to be used. A typical agent to use as a chelating agent is DMSA at a dose of 1000 mg, one hour after the first-morning urine. After taking the chelating agent, a urine collection is started for a set number of hours. Anywhere from 6 to

24 hours is sufficient to get accurate results.[37,38,39,40] Collecting all urine for 6 hours is just as adequate and much easier for the patient than 24 hours.

As a rule, we don't perform the provocative heavy metal test right away. Often, the test is run a few months after blood, saliva, and stool. The reason? The levels of "good" metals in the initial blood work need to be reviewed before running the heavy metal test. As we mobilize large amounts of "bad" metals and pass them into urine for testing, we are doing the same with "good" metals. If someone is quite low in RBC magnesium when the provocative heavy metal test is run, the further depletion of magnesium on the day of testing could cause heart palpitations and arrhythmias.[41] If the RBC magnesium level is low or on the lower end of the reference range at the time of initial blood work, spend a couple of months repleting the magnesium level with supplementation, retest to confirm correction to at least mid-range before doing the provocative heavy metal test.

FOOD SENSITIVITY TEST

Food can bother us in two ways: Immediate hypersensitivity reactions and delayed reactions. "Immediate hypersensitivity reactions involve IgA and IgE. Delayed reactions involve IgG."[32] However, IgG food testing can cause a heated conversation when talking with a more traditional western allopathic medical provider.

They argue against this form of testing despite much clinical experience and research backing up the value and the profound impact on the gut when these foods are eliminated. One piece of research was published in the British Medical Journal Open Gastroenterology in 2017.[42] It observed IgG testing and irritable bowel syndrome (IBS) patients. By eliminating foods identified on IgG testing as problematic, this hard-to-treat group of patients improved after only 4 weeks and were much better at 8 weeks. No other changes were made other than to stop eating some foods that tested positive on a simple IgG test.

Immediate hypersensitivity food reactions tend to be fast and dramatic. So fast, that the individual realizes they have an issue with a specific type of food or food group. Common IgE reactions include peanut allergies in children. If a child needs to go to the emergency room after eating a peanut, it is obvious they do not eat a peanut again. Common IgA reactions include people who get gassy and have diarrhea 10 minutes after consuming ice cream. This could be lactose intolerance or sugar in cow's milk dairy issue. But our biggest concern when it comes to AD is the proteins in foods, such as ones found in cow's milk dairy products. Thus, even lactose-free products should be avoided by someone with an AD. The typical tests performed for these immediate hypersensitivity reactions tend to be inaccurate.[43,44] Oftentimes, these include a skin analysis and blood work at a hospital or local testing lab. These tests may say a specific food result is negative, but the person has an adverse reaction every time they eat it. Alternatively, the test is positive, but the food does not cause immediate reactions after consumption. Often, the patient can determine what foods trouble them without the assistance of these tests.

However, foods can also bother us several days or even 3-4 weeks later. Better known as delayed hypersensitivity reactions, or IgG reactions, they do not cause the dramatic "hit" as in immediate hypersensitivity reactions. Thus, they won't send someone to the hospital. However, they tend to create a scenario where a person feels chronic inflammation and low-energy, or they feel like crud all the time, or their body is going haywire. They can't pinpoint a cause but attempt to address what they're eating. At this point, they might go a couple of weeks without eating certain foods and then assume it's not the food when they don't feel better, or they don't feel worse after consuming the food again. Albeit, during this process, they still haven't got "hit" from the last time they ate the food. They still haven't cleaned up all that chronic inflammation, so they still won't feel better. This is why it's crucial to test and not play the same guessing game as the patient.

Perhaps this dialogue regarding IgG food testing will go how the "no way an infection can cause stomach ulcers" debate went. We no longer think twice about the concept that H. Pylori bacterial infections of the stomach can cause ulcers. We also don't think twice about testing for and treating this infection. Also, the "leaky gut" debate has morphed into "intestinal permeability disorder." This continues despite all the data on the disruption of the intestinal tight junctions and its negative impact on gut function and chronic disease in general.

Just because something is not common knowledge yet, doesn't mean it's not real and important. An excellent example is the old "there is no reason to wash your hands between the time you did that autopsy and delivered that baby." This death-producing mindset persisted until Luweenhook developed the microscope in 1668 and bacteria were discovered in 1676.

Different lab companies offer assorted IgG testing kits. Some kits can test up to 500 foods. The most common test we start with is one that tests for 96 foods, grading each food 0-4. Not only do we know what is creating an issue, but also how much. You will find more information on the specific testing kits we use later in the book.

When it comes to AD, everyone with an autoimmune problem will have a delayed hypersensitivity reaction to wheat/gluten proteins and cows milk dairy proteins.[45] No exceptions. 62 proteins in wheat bother everyone at least a little bit. Everyone. Yet, in people with AD, the gut has not been able to clear the subtle injury quickly enough, and damage has accumulated over time—contributing to the development of the AD. The proteins in wheat (gluten being just one of them) and cow's milk dairy should always be eliminated from the diet, even if they do not show up positive on food sensitivity testing. Often, butter is okay because it is the protein that is problematic, not the fats. Butter is all fat and is the only food source for an essential nutrient for maintaining gut health. It is an important nutrient that is tested for on the digestive stool analysis tests: N-butyrate.

THE ELIMINATION DIET
(as an Alternative to the FST)

If for financial reasons, a patient can't do the FST, then a good alternative is an elimination diet. This is a one-page instruction sheet (see Figure 5). In the far left column are food categories. The middle column lists foods to include. On the far right, ones to exclude.

Category	Foods to Include	Foods to Exclude
Fruits Choose deeply colored, in season, organic and locally grown	Fresh or unsweetened frozen fruits Diluted unsweetened fruit juices	Oranges and dried fruits
Vegetables Choose deeply colored, in season, organic and locally grown	All fresh raw, steamed, sauteed, juice or roasted vegetables including sweet potatoes and yams	Corn, creamed vegetables, nightshades (such as tomatoes, white potatoes, egg plants, peppers, paprika, salsa, chili peppers, and cayenne chili powder)
Starch/Bread/Cereals	Rice, millet, quinoa, amaranth, teff flour, tapioca, buckwheat, "gluten free" oats	All gluten containing grains, wheat, barley, spelt, oat, kamut, rye, triticale
Legumes	All beans, peas, and lentils. Hummus is ok unless otherwise indicated	Soybeans, tofu, tempeh, soy milk, soy sauce, edamame, other soy products
Nuts and Seeds	Almonds, cashews, walnuts, brazil sesame (tahini), sunflower flax, pumpkin seeds. All butters made from these nuts/seeds are acceptable	Peanuts, peanut butter
Meats and Fish Choose low mercury fish, grass-fed lamb, hormone and antibiotic free poultry	All canned (water-packed), frozen or fresh low mercury fish. Chicken, turkey, wild game and lamb	Beef, pork, cold cuts, frankfurters, sausage, canned meats, eggs, shellfish
Dairy Products and Milk Substitutes	Milk substitutes such as rice milk, hemp milk, almond milk, and coconut milk	Milk, cheese, cottage cheese, cream, yogurt, butter, ice cream, frozen yogurt, "non-dairy creamers
Fats	For cooking: cold pressed olive oil, coconut oil, flaxseed oil, sunflower oil, sesame oil, walnut oil, pumpkin oil, or almond oil	Margarine, butter, shortening, processed or hydrogenated oils, mayonnaise spreads
Beverages	Filtered or distilled water, herbal teas, seltzer or mineral waters	Soda, soft drinks, alcoholic beverages, coffee, tea, caffeinated beverages
Herbs and Spices	All spices unless otherwise indicated. Vinegar is acceptable	Chocolate, ketchup, mustard, relish, chutney, soy sauce, teriyaki, tamari, other condiments

Figure 5

What I tell patients is, "the 'foods to exclude' column can't include every food a person might consume, so only eat the foods in the middle column." Indeed, everyone is unique; they may have some foods in the 'foods to include' that trouble them, even though most folks are okay. Yes, there will probably be foods in the 'to exclude' column that do not bother them. We are just playing the odds with an elimination diet intervention. It's not perfect, but it is a good option if a FST can't be used.

TREATMENT OPTIONS TO CONSIDER AT THE TIME OF FIRST VISIT

Even Before Lab Data is Available

Do not go where the path may lead, go instead where there is no path and leave a trail.

—Ralph Waldo Emerson

LOW DOSE NALTREXONE (LDN)

When naltrexone was first used, it was in relatively high doses (50-100mg daily). As such, it acts as an immunosuppressant. However, it was discovered that at low doses, naltrexone acts as an immunomodulator.[46] It rebalances the immune system, re-establishing the set-point.

At first, LDN was used most often in multiple sclerosis patients. But, as noted, all AD is the same disease– a 'poly-autoimmunity' that attacks various body parts. This fact made people wonder whether LDN could be used for all AD, and more recent studies have shown this appears to be the case. LDN could treat inflammatory bowel diseases such as ulcerative colitis and Crohn's disease, for example.

As an immune system modulator, LDN helps the upregulated and downregulated immune system issues in unison. It treats pain and inflammation and can help with weight loss. It also has a significant positive impact on brain function.

In adults, dosing of LDN can start at 1.5 mg at bedtime. Every week to two, the dose is increased by 1.5 mg until it reaches 4.5 mg. If, during the increasing dosage, a patient feels unwell, return to the last well-tolerated dose.

Seldom, someone may feel ill with a 1.5 mg dose. If this is the case, start with a 0.5 mg dose and wean up by 0.5mg every 1-2 weeks, until they are at 1.0 mg, if possible. In children, dosages of 0.1mg per kg of body weight have been used with success for at least six weeks, if not longer.

STRESS MANAGEMENT

Initiating daily stress relief exercise for at least 1-2 minutes a day is vital. Both, for its therapeutic impact, (the body heals better when it is not stuck in the "fight or flight" mode), and to make the patient understand right away this will be critical in their overall recovery.

There are many ways to create calm in the body. Meditation, music, deep breathing, repetitive prayer, body scanning, progressive muscle relaxation, yoga, tai chi, etc. There is a phone app called "Insight Timer" that many patients like and it's free. There is also "Inner Engineering," a yoga and meditation program offering CME credits through the Isha Foundation and the AMA. Please visit *www.DrDavidBilstrom.com/npadguide* for more details, including what can be achieved using music, based on the work of the music therapist Tim Ringgold. And of course, using Nature to heal.

AVOID CERTAIN PROTEINS

Aim for wheat/gluten-free and cow's milk dairy protein-free foods. Butter is ok.

When someone presents to you with an AD, they have a delayed hypersensitivity reaction to the proteins in wheat (gluten is just one of 62 proteins in wheat that create inflammation in the human gut) and cow's milk dairy proteins. Everyone is so unique, no one knows how much they bother each individual. However, it is obvious they disturb the patient to some degree.

If a patient has not tried to avoid wheat/gluten and cow's milk dairy proteins (at the same time) for at least four weeks before seeing you, this can be a good recommendation on their first visit. Then, wait to see what happens before proceeding with a food sensitivity test (FST).

If the patient returns to the second visit and says, "Holy cow! I feel much better after avoiding those two foods. I'm already 50-60-70-80% improved!" those may be the only proteins causing them trouble. Maybe they don't need the FST after all.

However, if they return and say, "I avoided those two things, but I don't feel much better," then other foods disturb them and a FST is needed—or, an elimination diet. If someone avoids foods they're sensitive to, they will feel much better, and this opens the window of opportunity for the body to correct everything. Including, in due course, all the food sensitivities except wheat/gluten. Once the body starts to "self-destruct," wheat/gluten will always need to be avoided.

More often than not, butter is ok. Butter is 99.99% fat and good fat. It is the proteins in certain foods that are so problematic for people with ADs. Not the fats or the carbs/sugars (although everyone becomes lactose intolerant sometime during their lifetime.)

We, as humans, are the only mammals who continue to consume milk after infancy. Thus, we sooner or later become intolerant of the sugar lactose that is in milk products. And, as I mentioned earlier, butter is the only food source of the essential short-chain fatty acid named n-butyrate. N-butyrate is so critical it is tested for in the digestive stool analysis. Don't cook with butter at high temperatures, as it denatures and becomes problematic. Use ghee if cooking at high temperatures. Add butter (ideally organic, non-GMO butter) to the food after it is cooked and just before consuming.

L-THEANINE

If someone has issues with anxiety, panic attacks, inability to sleep due to not being able to "turn their brain off" at the time of their first visit, consider starting them on L-theanine. L-theanine is an amino acid that becomes depleted with long-term, high levels of stress— being stuck in the "fight or flight" mode for a long time. Yet, the body cannot create calm without l-theanine. If someone is l-theanine depleted, they will feel calmer, and better overall, after getting started on this supplement.

Dosage: L-theanine at 1 capsule (100mg) in the AM and 2 capsules at HS (NuMedica). They may also use 1 capsule q3-4 hours prn for anxiety or insomnia. Max of 600 mg daily.

TEST INTERPRETATION

Life is very simple, but we insist on making it complicated.

—Confucius

BLOOD WORK: INTERPRETATION

Overview: Interpreting the data seen on the blood test results sheet

Every blood test report has three columns. The left-hand column is the test name. The middle column refers to the specific results for the patient. The right side is the reference range or the "normal range." Most practitioners treat the reference range as the ideal. Patients are often told, "Your results are in the reference range. You are normal and healthy." But, oftentimes the patient may reply, " I feel pretty crummy for someone whose labs say they are healthy. What's the deal?" The deal is, the reference range is not where the healthy people are, even though it is often treated that way. Testing labs get a lot of results from all the people tested. The distribution of the results looks like a bell-shaped curve. (see Figure 6)

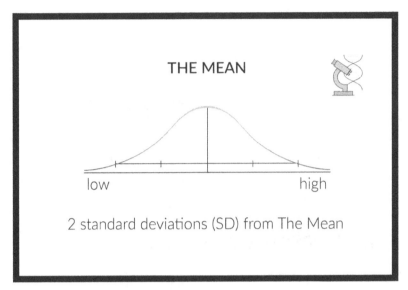

THE MEAN

low   high

2 standard deviations (SD) from The Mean

Figure 6

On the left is the lower end of the range and on the right is the higher end. Most results are in the middle. If we weigh 100 folks, some people are skinny and some are quite heavy; however, most are average.

The labs try to develop the reference range. In a perfect world, they would scour the thousands upon thousands of medical journals and identify the ideal physiologic range for optimal human health as it applies to every test run. Unfortunately, this takes a lot of work and it's not a perfect world. Instead, the labs use statistics. Next, and arbitrarily, they decide that all individuals who fall within 2 standard deviations from the mean (+/- 2 SD) will be within the reference range. By definition, 95% of all results, no matter what is being tested, will fall within 2 standard deviations from the mean.

But that doesn't account for who is being tested. It doesn't matter if it's a bunch of sick individuals, a group of healthy people, or a pack of baboons. It is just statistics; it doesn't determine what's healthy, it establishes what's common or "normal."

The question also comes down to who goes in to have their blood drawn. It's often the ones who feel so poorly, they had to see a medical practitioner. Thus, labs tend to test people who already feel unwell. When someone wants to feel robust, they may find a better value in knowing where they are compared to "healthy people" rather than all the folks who were so sick that they were tested. A person may, for example, like to know how they compare to individuals who climbed Mount Everest or became astronauts.

Because the reference range takes in 95% of the possible scores, when someone is flagged as being either high or low on a specific blood test, they know that out of 100, they're in the worst five. They failed this test. [They got an "F" on their test.] If they are not flagged, then they are not an "F" grade, but they are still left somewhere between a "D–" and an "A+". But no one wants a grade of a "C" or a "D" when it comes to their health. People generally want to be in the "A" range, which is where human biochemistry and physiology work the best.[32]

If an individual's test results are not in the physiologic range, we need to discover how to make them feel healthy again. Thus, how do we know where these physiologic ranges are? From the hundreds, if not thousands of studies about every item we test. And yes, tests for lab ranges have been performed on astronauts and folks who climbed Mount Everest.

Included in this chapter will be not only the names of the tests that need to be run but also the physiological ranges. Because new data is always coming out, these ranges will likely change as we fine-tune things over the next few years. A general rule, however, is that if something is good (such as vitamin D, RBC magnesium, RBC zinc), the upper end of the range is best. If something is bad (such as reverse

T3 in the setting of hypothyroidism) the lower end of the reference range is perfect.

This is also why you will see different reference ranges being used by different labs. You can tell a lot about the particular population being tested by a certain lab company by the reference ranges produced. For example, a fasting blood sugar range of 70 to 100 differs from one that goes up to 110. The people in that community tend to have higher fasting blood sugars than those in another population. The same principle applies to a lab with a vitamin D range of 10 to 50 compared with a 20 to 80 range.[32]

The ideal levels of the most important blood work tests

WBC (within the reference range is sufficient).
Scores below the range are consistent with a down-regulated immune system. The low WBC is partly the cause of chronic infections. If the score is high, be suspicious of existing chronic infections (although be suspicious of chronic infections even before seeing this test result).

Fasting insulin and blood sugar (BS)
    Insulin (4-6).
    Blood sugar (Ideally low 70's or at least ≤ 84).

Note: As insulin resistance begins, fasting BS increases, creating inflammation and wild swings in BS. The pancreas should respond by making more insulin. However, because of insulin resistance, the insulin still does not get much bang for its effort, and fasting BS continues to climb. Eventually, the pancreas may have been so overworked that the insulin levels become too low. For every one-point above 84, the patient has a 6% chance of diabetes in the next 10 years. Thus, an individual can be well within the range and still be almost guaranteed diabetes. Unless you fix them, of course.

Liver enzymes SGPT and SGOT
(within the reference range is sufficient for these)
If the score is high, the liver is inflamed; "hepatitis", even if not a typical Hep A or Hep B—is still inflammation of the liver. Of course, if the situation warrants further testing regarding the cause of the elevated LFTs, please do all that is required. If LFTs are low, the liver cannot create important proteins such as glutathione—the most potent free radical scavenger the body can make.

GFR (>90)
This is often low when a patient with an AD first presents to you. The kidneys are miserable. The inflammation affecting the body as a whole is also hurting the kidneys. Is the patient in the 60-89 range? Consider just watching to see if it corrects itself as you address the big picture. More often than not, it will. If it doesn't improve, or if it is in the moderate kidney damage range (30-59), consider NAC (N-Acetylcysteine). If <30, consult the Renal service and start NAC 2 twice per day.

Note: consider starting NAC at one capsule daily and increase to one capsule twice a day after a week if the patient seems quite toxic. In the setting of severe toxic overload, they could experience unpleasant detox reactions. However, this is uncommon with oral treatment. It is more frequent with the use of IV glutathione if the gut has not had a chance to heal yet by avoiding offending foods, etc.

Vitamin D (70-80 though some say 80-90 is better).
Vitamin D is not a genuine vitamin, but a prohormone. Vitamin D gets "bad press" with its importance minimized or even questioned. The 11,000+ scientific journal articles on how vitamin D works biochemically and physiologically regarding health maintenance and reversing disease disagree.

Some Vitamin D research findings:

- Vitamin D levels 50 or greater during pregnancy decrease the risk of the child getting multiple sclerosis by 50%.[47]
- 2000 IU per day during an infant's first 12 months of life decreases their risk of Type 1 diabetes by almost 90%.[48]
- Vitamin D levels ≥ 60 decrease breast cancer risk in women by 82%.[49]
- Vitamin D deficiency accounts for premature deaths from the following types of cancer: colon, breast, ovarian, and prostate.[50]
- Vitamin D receptor activity in the gut plays a vital role in inflammatory bowel disease and chronic disease in general.[51]

Optimizing vitamin D levels is important in maintaining overall health, and levels can be optimized faster when compared to others, such as oral iron. Most people need at least 5000-10,000 IU per day of vitamin D. It's imperative to monitor their levels to keep them in an optimal range.

Vitamin D is not to be used for a time and then discontinued. Due to various factors, nearly everyone has lower vitamin D levels than ideal, unless they are on long-term vitamin D supplementation.[52] Once in a while, someone may only need 1000-2000 IU per day. (Low vitamin D can also cause low back pain among other problems, so it's fundamental.)

Note: Vitamin D optimization is always begun at the first follow-up visit once the 25 OH vitamin D level is known.

Ferritin (~100)
Ferritin levels being too high without being on iron supplementation also suggests an inability to clear toxic elements. If ferritin levels are low, oxygen cannot be carried to the tissues in our bodies.[53] If the level is below the reference range, order IV iron once a week for two weeks, to faster replete this deficiency. It can be frustratingly slow to

correct low ferritin using oral supplementation. Many insurances will cover IV iron infusions (feraheme). My habit is not to ask the patient to pay out of pocket if it's not covered by insurance. Albeit, even if the preauthorization is done and insurance says they will pay, the patient should make sure they have paid enough of their deductible to avoid the high cost of the iron IVs.

B12 (≥ 800-900)
Homocysteine (5-7)
Homocysteine levels tend to indicate B vitamin status. "When homocysteine is high, B vitamin levels are low."[32] Levels can also be impacted by other issues, such as kidney disease. B vitamins are vital to our well-being, so this is an essential test to run. Consider all the diseases that are more likely to occur when homocysteine levels are too high: heart attack, stroke, cancer, osteoporosis, mood issues, Alzheimer's, diabetes, gut dysfunction, and ADs, to name just a few.[54,55,56,57,58,59,60,61,62,63,64] B vitamins are critical for nerve health and neuropathic pain issues almost always require B vitamins for healing.[65,66,67]

Note: The methylation status of B vitamins is vital. Often, they must be fully activated, fully methylated B vitamins. There are many reasons we can't stick a methyl group on the inactive B vitamins from food in the 21st Century. The names of the activated B vitamins are, for example:

- B12: methylcobalamin; not cyanocobalamin
- B6: pyridoxal — 5' — phosphate
- B2: riboflavin — 5' — phosphate
- Folate: methyltetrahydrofolic acid

Also, fully activated B complexes that include trimethylglycine are beneficial. Its common name is betaine and it is a great methyl donor. We need to methylate fat-soluble toxins so they can turn into water-soluble ones to clear them from the body. We should methylate our DNA to shut down bad genes and activate good genes to optimize epigenetic influence on health.[68]

Note: As homocysteine levels improve, point it out to the patient and let them know how wonderful it is they are correcting high homocysteine for the above reasons. No one wants the diseases associated with high homocysteine levels.

RBC Magnesium (6.0-6.4 on most reference ranges)
The reference range runs from 4.2-6.4. Occasionally, a different range will be used but a person should still be at the upper end.

RBC Zinc (>12)

Thyroid labs. TSH, free T4, free T3, reverse T3, TPO ABs, and thyroglobulin ABs

The thyroid is called, 'the great mimicker,' as disruption can present with a variety of symptoms. Whenever someone has multiple organ system involvements, thyroid hormone issues are a likely contributor.

The thyroid's involvement in chronic disease and AD is often missed because not enough thyroid tests are run in blood work and the interpretation of the results is less than optimal. Free T4 is the primary hormone made by the thyroid itself, but it is a rather inactive hormone. TSH (thyroid-stimulating hormone) explains T4's status. Thus TSH is not a great test. When TSH is low, this suggests too much T4. When TSH is high, this suggests we need more T4. Needing more T4 implies that the thyroid is not keeping up with T4 production needs. When TSH is high and T4 is low, a T4 medicine may be used because the person's thyroid is not making enough. At this point, the person has been identified as a "poor thyroid producer."

Not so long ago, T4 dosing was based on symptom resolution. Start low and go slow. Increase the dosage in increments until the person feels their best. Doses for optimal symptom resolution were 200-300 mcg per day, on average. All this changed in the late 1970s when the TSH test was invented. Dosing of T4 medication began to be based on TSH levels. Doses dropped almost at once to 100 to 150 micrograms daily. Folks were left under-treated, and many more people will continue to suffer if dosing is based on TSH levels alone.[69]

However, something different occurred in the last two to three decades. It is no longer enough to determine if someone has poor thyroid production. Many people these days are poor thyroid converters. Or, they are poor thyroid producers and converters. Someone may have optimal T4 and TSH levels on testing, but cannot convert the inactive T4 into the more active and usable free T3. Instead, they convert the free T4 to the inactive thyroid hormone called reverse T3 (rT3).[69] Excessive rT3 will block the T3 receptors on every cell of the body so much, the available free T3 will not have a chance to act.

The people with ideal levels of TSH and free T4 without thyroid medication may be poor T4 converters. As a result, all their symptoms may point to low thyroid. What causes poor thyroid conversion? Vitamin and mineral deficiencies, stress, the stress hormone cortisol, toxicity, eating too many carbs, and not enough protein—just to list a few.

We are living in the 21st-century; everyone is vitamin and mineral-deficient. The nutrient content of food is depleted. Our guts have a tough time absorbing nutrients even with high-quality foods. People tend to eat too many carbohydrates and not enough protein. The typical way for most people is the "SAD" diet—the Standard American Diet, and it has negative consequences. Folks here in the U.S. spend so much money on over-the-counter products for diarrhea, constipation, reflux, bloating, and similar ailments. An estimated 10-15% of individuals worldwide suffer from irritable bowel syndrome.[70] Everyone is stressed out. Everyone is toxic. A 2006 study of umbilical cord blood discovered that every baby is born with mercury, flame retardants, pesticides, and herbicides already in their systems.[71] This goes back to epigenetics. To optimize epigenetics before a woman (or man) conceives, toxins should be cleared from their system. When a woman still has many environmental toxins at conception, the toxins will cross the placenta during gestation. Thus, the high levels of toxicity even at birth!

In a poor thyroid converter, it can be challenging if not impossible to get the best control of all the thyroid-related symptoms with T4 thyroid medication. They convert the T4 to reverse T3, rather than free T3. Desiccated thyroid medications can be an excellent option in this situation. T3-only products can also be an excellent option. Due to the short half-life of the T3 products (4-6 hours) they are usually dosed two times a day. This still leaves a lot of time within 24-hours when the active T3 levels will be less than optimal. If possible, using a compounded, sustained action T3 medication (c-E4M T3) can be the best option. This will maintain consistent T3 levels.

For example, when poor thyroid conversion is an issue, you could convert 100 micrograms of a T4 product to 60 mg of a desiccated thyroid product. 50 micrograms of a T4 product converts to 30 mg of a desiccated product, and this drops the level of T4, effectively dropping the level of rT3. Desiccated products already have T3, so the free T3 levels can remain the same, or rise to ideal levels.

Newer research suggests that people with autoimmune thyroid disease, such as Hashimoto's Thyroiditis, might want to avoid the use of porcine-based desiccated thyroid medicines. Instead, they may benefit from the use of a compounded non-porcine equivalent to the desiccated products.

Note: A handy way to get a sense of how much thyroid issues impact someone's multiple organ system dysfunctions is "The signs and symptoms of low thyroid." (see Figure 7 and visit *www.DrDavidBilstrom.com/npadguide* for a downloadable copy) This is a list of symptoms that may occur if the thyroid is low. I've been using it for years.

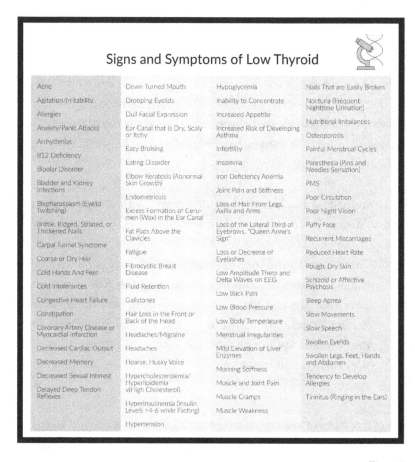

Signs and Symptoms of Low Thyroid

Acne	Down Turned Mouth	Hypoglycemia	Nails That are Easily Broken
Agitation/Irritability	Drooping Eyelids	Inability to Concentrate	Nocturia (Frequent Nighttime Urination)
Allergies	Dull Facial Expression	Increased Appetite	
Anxiety/Panic Attacks	Ear Canal that is Dry, Scaly or Itchy	Increased Risk of Developing Asthma	Nutritional Imbalances
Arrhythmias			Osteoporosis
B12 Deficiency	Easy Bruising	Infertility	Painful Menstrual Cycles
Bipolar Disorder	Eating Disorder	Insomnia	Paresthesia (Pins and Needles Sensation)
Bladder and Kidney Infections	Elbow Keratosis (Abnormal Skin Growth)	Iron Deficiency Anemia	PMS
Blepharospasm (Eyelid Twitching)	Endometriosis	Joint Pain and Stiffness	Poor Circulation
	Excess Formation of Cerumen (Wax) in the Ear Canal	Loss of Hair From Legs, Axilla and Arms	Poor Night Vision
Brittle, Ridged, Striated, or Thickened Nails	Fat Pads Above the Clavicles	Loss of the Lateral Third of Eyebrows, "Queen Anne's Sign"	Puffy Face
Carpal Tunnel Syndrome			Recurrent Miscarriages
Coarse or Dry Hair	Fatigue	Loss or Decrease of Eyelashes	Reduced Heart Rate
Cold Hands And Feet	Fibrocystic Breast Disease	Low Amplitude Theta and Delta Waves on EEG	Rough, Dry Skin
Cold Intolerances	Fluid Retention		Schizoid or Affective Psychosis
Congestive Heart Failure	Gallstones	Low Back Pain	Sleep Apnea
Constipation	Hair Loss in the Front or Back of the Head	Low Blood Pressure	Slow Movements
Coronary Artery Disease or Myocardial Infarction		Low Body Temperature	Slow Speech
	Headaches/Migraine	Menstrual Irregularities	Swollen Eyelids
Decreased Cardiac Output	Headaches	Mild Elevation of Liver Enzymes	Swollen Legs, Feet, Hands and Abdomen
Decreased Memory	Hoarse, Husky Voice	Morning Stiffness	
Decreased Sexual Interest	Hypercholesterolemia/ Hyperlipidemia (High Cholesterol)	Muscle and Joint Pain	Tendency to Develop Allergies
Delayed Deep Tendon Reflexes		Muscle Cramps	Tinnitus (Ringing in the Ears)
	Hyperinsulinemia (Insulin Levels >4-6 while Fasting)	Muscle Weakness	
	Hypertension		

Figure 7

Often, a patient is asked to review the list and circle all symptoms that apply. The more symptoms they highlight, the more the thyroid is impacting the person's overall health. It will also suggest the potential positive impact of correcting thyroid issues.

- TSH (<2.0)
- Free T4 (In adults ≥ 1.0. In teenagers ≥1.2. In children ≥1.4)
- Free T3 (In adults ≥ 3.5 though some people feel great at 3.1-3.2. In teenagers ≥4.0. In children ≥ 4.2)
- Reverse T3 (8-10 with the typical range being 8-25)
- Thyroglobulin ABs and TPO ABs (Zero)

Note: there is never a good reason for the immune system to attack another body part—even a little bit. Thus, zero for both of these types of thyroid antibodies is best. Even ≥ 1.0 is bad for the thyroglobulin ABs. Sometimes, the ranges for TPO ABs say <35 is ok. Although zeros are my favorite.

If the individual has never been diagnosed with an autoimmune thyroid disease before, then explain what it means.

> "It is never a good idea to attack our body parts. As we repair the big picture, it should decrease, with the goal of reaching zero. We can use these numbers as feedback on how well we are doing with fixing the immune system; rebalancing the immune system as a whole. Not only getting rid of the upregulated autoimmune disease, but also the infection and cancer risk."[32]

The early stages of autoimmune thyroid disease have often started by the time someone comes in with an AD. Sometimes, it's full-blown Hashimoto's. If the antibodies are present, but not high enough to be out-of-the-range high, I just say they have an early autoimmune thyroid process beginning. You could tell the patient they have Hashimoto's but they are probably overwhelmed already, putting another AD name on it could add more stress but it won't change the management.

It doesn't matter what name a disease is given when it comes to reversing autoimmune problems. It is much more important to know why people have whatever it is we are trying to normalize. When we know the "why," we can fix almost anything, no matter what the diagnosis.

DHEA-S (women >150. Men >350)

This hormone is created by the adrenal gland and impacted by chronic stress. DHEA levels will drop if a body/someone has been stuck in stress mode for too long (and cortisol is always high.) If DHEA levels drop, this will cause the chronically elevated cortisol to start crashing. DHEA will need to be started right away, to prevent cortisol from crashing and begin the ticking time bomb for worse health issues such as heart attacks, strokes, cancer, and diabetes.

DHEA crashing is itself a major part of what causes the ticking time bomb of the cortisol crash. Low DHEA is a significant risk factor for heart attacks and strokes.[72,73] Further, it is difficult for a body to create anything that is protein-based without DHEA, including neurotransmitters, hormones, enzymes, cell walls, etc.[74] So much of our body is protein-based, including proteins made by DNA, for proper cell functioning.

Pregnenolone (>100) The 'brain hormone'

Pregnenolone converts to progesterone as part of the steroidogenic hormone production cascade. But without adequate DHEA, pregnenolone can "shunt" to DHEA and then convert to testosterone and estrogen.

Later, we will review a workaround when it comes to getting a patient to optimal levels of the hormones progesterone, testosterone, estradiol, and estrone without having to use these downstream hormones. This involves understanding the wonderful steroidogenic hormone production cascade.

CoQ10 (≥ 1.6)
The major source of CoQ10 is biosynthesis.[75] CoQ10 fuels the mitochondria needed to make ATP and powers up the cell. It's significant because the muscles, brain, thyroid, heart, and intestines contain much of the body's CoQ10, and they require ATP to function. When an individual has chronic health issues, they find it challenging to maintain adequate production of CoQ10. Significant issues in these tissues, or overall fatigue in general, may suggest the need for CoQ10 supplementation.

However, the body is amazing and many folks will start to make more CoQ10 when their body starts to heal. In other words, they may not need supplementation long term. Even though it has been said that most people over the age of 40 will have difficulty making adequate CoQ10 to "power-up," folks much older can still eventually produce adequate CoQ10.

Note: If a person has a history of cardiovascular disease, they may benefit from levels of ≥ 3.5. If Parkinson's Disease, ≥ 4.0.

Infections. (EBV titers absent or low. All other infection titers absent)
Chronic infections are common drivers of AD and are related to many health issues including chronic pain. Some infections, such as a cold or pneumonia, invade our bodies and we know it right away. We hope the symptoms are short-term. Sometimes, however, they create immediate reactions (such as the Epstein-Barr virus and mononucleosis) but can remain dormant and create new problems years or decades later. Thus, getting mononucleosis more than doubles the risk of multiple sclerosis later in life.[76,77]

Once the immune system has become dysregulated enough, it is not just one bug or one infection, it's multiple. If one bug gets inside, more can get in. Often, it's a combination of viruses, bacteria, fungi, and mycoplasma. At this point, a broad-spectrum antimicrobial is needed to clear all the infections at once. These infections can be found in the blood test and/or the stool test and they tend to be stubborn to clear. Molds will usually take at least 3 months but mycoplasma can take 6, 9, 12 months, or longer to clear.

When it comes to mycoplasma, don't be fooled. Antibiotics may look like a reasonable option to clear mycoplasma because it is sensitive to these agents. Of course, antibiotics won't clear viruses or fungi. It might look even more tempting to use an antibiotic against mycoplasma given they do not have cell walls and can never develop a resistance to an antibiotic. Because mycoplasma surrounds itself with a biofilm, it is hard to destroy. An antibiotic used for several months would still not clear it. And by then the gut has become so disrupted all sorts of new issues have developed. I've seen people with rheumatoid arthritis who were on antibiotics twice a day for almost ten years, trying to clear the identified mycoplasma. Their joint pain lessened by 70-80% but their gut became so dysfunctional from the antibiotics 4-5 other autoimmune diseases emerged in the process. Moreover, antibiotics don't clear fungi or viruses.

Powerful, long-duration antimicrobials are available. One such product is pH Structured Silver Solution—a silver formulation that can be effective at low doses.[78,79,80] It can be used indefinitely and at the doses/frequency needed.

People have used colloidal silver to treat infections for a long time. Silver is a great antimicrobial, but colloidal silver is not potent and must be used in high doses. However, doses are so high they can never be used for long durations. It can produce toxic levels to the point that skin turns blue.

"Silver preparations formulated like the pH Structured Silver Solution are able to work well at low doses."[32] People can take more than required every day, and use it for many decades, but never reach toxic levels. Mycoplasma creates pain, brain, and thyroid issues. Therefore, the patient can use the pH Structured Silver Solution until the mycoplasma infection is gone. When will that time come? When the patient no longer has pain or brain symptoms, and the autoimmune thyroid antibodies begin to resolve.

After the brain and pain issues are cleared, the patient may say they feel even 70-80% better overall. Thus, the chronic infections are probably gone, including mycoplasma. Then instruct the patient to discontinue the pH Structured Silver Solution and watch what happens. If they still feel just as well, then the infections have been cleared, and (fingers crossed), the immune system dysregulation has been corrected enough the infections will never return. However, if they stop the pH Structured Silver Solution and feel worse (usually this begins within 2-5 days of discontinuation), it should be resumed for another two months before they stop again. This process will continue until the patient feels just as well as without it.

Another broad-spectrum antimicrobial that can be very effective in the face of multiple chronic infections is a plant-based product called Biocidin. The first type is Liposomal Biocidin for systemic infections (not accompanied by gut infections). The other is Advanced Liquid Biocidin used for gut infections, or when the gut infections are accompanied by systemic infections. The Biocidin products are quick to kill bugs. Begin with small doses, increasing them in increments every few days. The goal is to reach the full dose and stay there until they feel 70-80% better. It is common to get die-off reactions, or Herzheimer's reactions, as the dose is increased. Thus, I recommend the Biocidin products along with a product called "GI Detox." GI Detox is a combination of charcoal and clay used to bind up the toxins released. As the dose of the Biocidin products is increased, if the patient feels worse (the die-off/Herzheimer's reaction), decrease the dose to the last one the patient tolerated, wait 3-5 days and increase the dose again. The Biocidin needs to be dosed three times a day and the GI Detox two times a day. They should be taken on an empty stomach, separate from each other, away from food and other supplements/medications. On the other hand, the pH Structured Silver Solution can be taken once a day and it doesn't matter when— making it a simpler regimen to follow.

Note: Epstein Barr Virus (EBV): Because most folks (perhaps 80% of all Americans) have been exposed to EBV sometime in their life, almost everyone produces some ABs against EBV. Thus, titers are positive. Yet, they don't necessarily indicate an active EBV infection. It denotes their immune system is familiar with EBV and has antibodies if the EBV invades again. However, if any of the titers reported have numbers so elevated the testing lab doesn't count that high (such as >600), then my concern is that EBV is creating issues. If two of the EBV titers are reported as greater than the set number determined by the lab, I am very concerned.

Note: All the other infections tested: If AB titers are positive, there is an active infection that must be cleared with long-term use of an antimicrobial such as the pH Structured Silver Solution.

Note: It is tough to find infections on standard blood work because tests look for antibodies produced by the immune system against a specific microorganism. The chronic infections involved in autoimmune disease are good at hiding from the immune system. The immune system might not even realize they have entered, so it does not produce antibodies, even though the "bug" is creating issues. Sometimes, the immune system is so disrupted, it doesn't have the energy to make antibodies anymore.

SPECIAL SECTION ON THE SEX HORMONES INTERPRETATION

Estradiol (Women 80-100. Men 20-40)

Estrone (Women ~30. Men <5-10)

Progesterone (Women ≥ 5-10. Men ~1-2)

Total testosterone (Women 40-60. Men 800-1100)

Free testosterone (Women 3-9. Men 200-300)

SHBG: sex hormone-binding globulin (~30)

Note: Some labs report free testosterone levels with the decimal point moved over one spot. On these ranges, free testosterone levels for men should be 20-30.

It is imperative to recognize that estrogen dominance (too much estrogen in relation to progesterone) is a significant issue with women and a huge driver of AD and disease in general. Estrogen dominance is one reason why 80% of individuals with ADs are women. For men, low testosterone is a significant contributor to chronic disease and can be the sole cause of back and neck pain, for example.[81,82]

When it comes to hormone restoration therapy, some hormones can be taken orally while others should only be used topically. Estrogen should never be taken orally. Any oral estrogen, no matter if it's bioidentical or non-bioidentical, will have a negative impact on gut function and other bodily functions.[83,84] Also, estrogen taken orally produces toxic byproducts as it passes through the liver.

Ideally, topical estrogen for women should be compounded BiEst 80/20. A ratio of 80% estriol and 20% estradiol. When using bio-identical hormone restoration therapy of any kind, think of the mantra, "start low and go slow." A reasonable starting dose of BiEst 80/20 could be 0.5 mg of a daily use topical cream.

Why is it important to use estriol and not just estradiol alone? Estriol is the weakest of the three estrogens the body produces but does about 80% of estrogen's work. Estriol has many functions in the body, but it is inefficient to prevent cardiovascular disease and keep bones strong alone; thus the 20% estradiol.

Estradiol is powerful enough to lower cardiovascular risk and improve bone health but can excessively convert into estrone.[85] Great caution should be exercised with topical estradiol in patch form because it tends to convert excessively to estrone and thus has a negative impact on the body.

Excess estrone is problematic for several reasons including its impact on breast tissue health. Breast tissue has two types of estrogen receptors: Type "A" and "B." A is called the "accelerator" and B is called the "brake." Too much accelerator without being well balanced with the brake is bad for breast tissue health. Estriol stimulates the "A" and "B" receptors at a 1:3 ratio, which is a lot more "brake" than "accelerator." Estradiol at a 1:1 ratio results in equal stimulation. But, estrone stimulates at a 5:1 ratio. That's five times more accelerator than brake. Keeping the percent of estradiol low, and letting estriol do much of the estrogen work, helps to avoid excessive conversion of estradiol to estrone.

Another appropriate dose could be BiEst 50/50. This may be better for someone transitioning from an oral product to a topical bioidentical product. The oral products have an excessive estrogen effect on the body. The body will be "dumping" estrogen as fast as it can for 6, 9, 12 months or longer. Thus, a higher dose and potentially the BiEst 50/50 may be needed to counter this until the body has cleared the estrogen "excess" and starts to detoxify the estrogens at more normal rates. Then, the dose can be lowered and the BiEst 50/50 be changed to BiEst 80/20. Remember that BiEst needs to be compounded.

There are many advantages to compounding. One big advantage is that doses can be individualized for each patient's exact needs. Often, with topically administered agents, symptom changes will begin after four to eight weeks. Retesting should be done after 12 weeks. Dosages can then be modified as needed. Ideally, when using topical bioidentical estrogen therapy (or any other topical bioidentical hormone therapy) saliva testing should be done. Blood levels will tend to underestimate the true levels of hormones in the system.[86]

Estrogen should always be used with progesterone. They work together in more than one way. For example, progesterone produces strong bones, while estrogen prevents bone loss. Also, estrogen tends to irritate breast tissue while progesterone protects it. When using estrogen, it's crucial to also use progesterone to protect the breast. This is also true for estrogen dominance and its negative impact on autoimmune disease prevention or reversal.[87]

Testosterone
Another hormone never to take orally is testosterone. Bio-identical testosterone is an option for both men and women. Injections can be a great option for men. However, methyltestosterone (non-bio-identical) is the sole commercially available testosterone for women and should be avoided due to the risk of liver cancer.[88]

When treating women, testosterone should always be taken with estrogen, and estrogen should always be taken with progesterone. Taking testosterone without estrogen will negatively impact a woman's cardiovascular health.

Topical testosterone dosing for women can start at 0.5 mg of cream and go up slowly. Topical dosing for men can start at 10mg.

IM testosterone for men is best in the lateral quadriceps muscle, 1-2 times a week. Advantages of IM include dosing once-a-week and no concerns regarding insufficient transdermal absorption. Topical use also comes with the risk of transferring testosterone to others through contact. Injectables are covered by most insurance. If injectables are not an option, a topical cream is superior to patches when it comes to absorption.

SHBG.
This will tend to go up when someone has too much of one hormone compared to other hormones. Remember the hormone symphony? The body is protecting you from the hormone imbalance. This is seen almost universally in the presence of estrogen dominance. The body is protecting a woman from excess estrogens.

SALIVA CORTISOL: INTERPRETATION
(See Figure 8)

Cortisol, the "stress hormone", should start at its highest levels in the morning and decrease as the day progresses, hitting its lowest point at bedtime. With this progression of cortisol throughout the day, we can fall asleep easily and nothing should wake us up overnight. We get wonderful restorative sleep, with no pain, no bladder, no noise waking us in the middle of the night. Nothing. So peaceful that some call it the 'sleep of the dead' for lack of a better term. When this happens, we wake up feeling great; energized, and refreshed. We can jump out of bed, no coffee needed, and feel prepared to do it all over again.

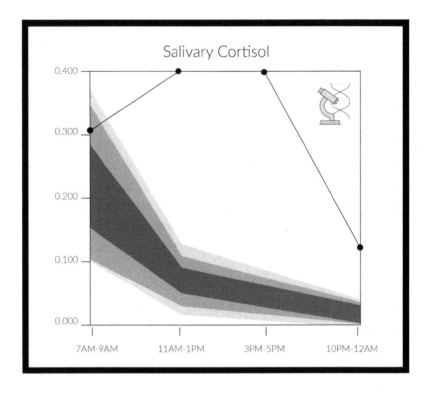

Figure 8

Almost every single person with an AD will have cortisol issues. Many of them may even deal with the complete opposite rhythm; low energy all day but then cannot shut down at night. Some describe it as feeling "tired and wired".

Cortisol is designed to go up and down many times a day. Stress is stress to the body. It doesn't matter if it is emotional, physical, spiritual, or biochemical. Driving home in a winter storm, "white-knuckling" the steering wheel is emotional stress. Kicking a chair leg while wearing open-toed shoes is physical stress. But if the stress someone has experienced is too great, or lasts too long, then the hormone cortisol can go way up and get stuck in the "on" position.. This is a perpetual state of the "flight or fight" mode, or the "life or death" mode. It's never good to hang out in the "A bear is chasing me trying to kill me" mode when no bear is chasing you.

When the body has high levels of cortisol at every time tested during the day, this is referred to as Stage one adrenal fatigue.[89] "These terms and concepts have been described in the scientific literature for many decades."[32] The reference listed above is from the British Medical Journal, from 1950!

The hormone DHEA, like cortisol, needs to stay at an ideal level, or even be temporarily increased, to let the person continue 'running from the bear,' even when they do not feel well. If a bear is in pursuit, you want to keep running. Stop running and your body thinks you are dead, so it acts accordingly. Yet, imagine if the individual runs 24 hours a day, seven days a week, day after day, month after month? The body can't keep up and they will feel worse over time.

In due course, after running from the bear long enough and getting sicker over time, the body/cortisol just can't continue. It's worn out. Cortisol levels start to crash. Being so sick for so long that cortisol levels crash is a bad place for a person with AD. However, at times, this cortisol crash is also a last-ditch effort by the body to heal: to save the brain from further deterioration. The most problematic areas of the brain are the hippocampus, hypothalamus, prefrontal cortex, and amygdala.[90]

It is the long-term high cortisol levels that create an immunosuppressed state, which allows the infections to establish themselves in the body.

Stage two adrenal fatigue means that one out of the four cortisol test results is lower than the ideal but the others are still high.[89] When two or more are low, it's reached stage three. The worst possibility occurs when someone has crashed all four times in a day. At this point, there is likely a "time bomb" that started ticking for issues like a heart attack, stroke, cancer, and diabetes.

Some newer terms that better reflect what is happening in the body: Hypercortisolism refers to when all levels are high; hypocortisolism refers to when all are low; mixed cortisolism refers to when some levels are low and some high.

For correctly interpreting the cortisol status, the status of the DHEA (or DHEA-S on blood testing) will disclose if the person is or isn't crashing. When cortisol first goes up and stays in the fight or flight mode, DHEA levels go up and keep the person going, even if they do not feel their best.

When test results show DHEA levels as too low (not in the middle of the green zone or higher), **even if cortisol levels are still too high**, cortisol will also crash. This is when I say to the patient, "Oh no, we need to stop this cortisol from crashing. We hate ticking time bombs."

This is when a medical practitioner running the test can be fooled. I see it all the time when someone has gone to a practitioner who runs the saliva cortisol and DHEA test but isn't great at interpreting the results. If crashing cortisol levels are near the sweet spot in the middle of the cortisol green zone, you might be tempted to say, "Despite the AD and all your health issues, cortisol looks pretty good so we don't need to do anything for your cortisol." This is a big mistake; a critical mistake.

Without starting someone on adrenal adaptogens to address the cortisol issues, nothing else you do will have the expected impact. The person with an AD will never feel as well as they should. The crashed DHEA levels are a sign that the cortisol is dropping as well.

On their way from high to low, they were just passing the green zone when the test was run.

I have seen people who were told their cortisol levels looked fine even though they were already a little bit lower than ideal.

Cortisol levels are never low unless a person has been in the 'up' position for a long time. If even one cortisol result is low, they are crashing. Don't be fooled.

People in their mid-teens and younger can usually reset their cortisol without using an adrenal adaptogen. They still need to do daily relaxation exercises, but can reset their cortisol by addressing the physical "bears", like the vitamin deficiencies, infections, gut issues, etc… After the mid-teens, everyone needs to address the biggest bear of all (cortisol), to turn everything around. They need adrenal adaptogens or great, daily relaxation activities. Almost always, they need both.

DIGESTIVE STOOL ANALYSIS: INTERPRETATION

(See Figure 9)

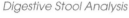

Digestive Stool Analysis

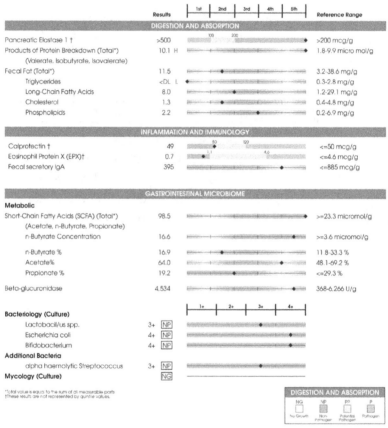

	Results	1st	2nd	3rd	4th	5th	Reference Range
DIGESTION AND ABSORPTION							
Pancreatic Elastase 1 †	>500						>200 mcg/g
Products of Protein Breakdown (Total*)	10.1 H						1.8-9.9 micro mol/g
(Valerate, Isobutyrate, Isovalerate)							
Fecal Fat (Total*)	11.5						3.2-38.6 mg/g
Triglycerides	<DL L						0.3-2.8 mg/g
Long-Chain Fatty Acids	8.0						1.2-29.1 mg/g
Cholesterol	1.3						0.4-4.8 mg/g
Phospholipids	2.2						0.2-6.9 mg/g
INFLAMMATION AND IMMUNOLOGY							
Calprotectin †	49						<=50 mcg/g
Eosinophil Protein X (EPX)†	0.7						<=4.6 mcg/g
Fecal secretory IgA	395						<=885 mcg/g
GASTROINTESTINAL MICROBIOME							
Metabolic							
Short-Chain Fatty Acids (SCFA) (Total*)	98.5						>=23.3 micromol/g
(Acetate, n-Butyrate, Propionate)							
n-Butyrate Concentration	16.6						>=3.6 micromol/g
n-Butyrate %	16.9						11.8-33.3 %
Acetate%	64.0						48.1-69.2 %
Propionate %	19.2						<=29.3 %
Beta-glucuronidase	4.534						368-6.266 U/g

		1+	2+	3+	4+	
Bacteriology (Culture)						
Lactobacil/us spp.	3+ NP					
Escherichia coli	4+ NP					
Bifidobacterium	4+ NP					
Additional Bacteria						
alpha haemolytic Streptococcus	3+ NP					
Mycology (Culture)	NG					

*Total value is equal to the sum of all measurable parts
†These results are not represented by quintile values.

DIGESTION AND ABSORPTION			
NG	NP	po	P
☐	☐	☐	☐
No Growth	Non-Pathogen	Potential Pathogen	Pathogen

Figure 9

Pancreatic Elastase (>500)

This is an important protein generated by the pancreas. It is crucial to know if the pancreas can still produce this protein in optimal amounts by the time you see the patient. It can drop for many reasons, including when the pancreas has been overworking to make insulin when insulin resistance has been present for a while.[91] The insulin resistance may have been there for so long that levels have dropped below ideal and the patient is transitioning from "prediabetes" to full-blown diabetes.

Note: If levels are <500, start the patient on specific supplements.

Fecal fats, fecal protein products, and possibly carbohydrates (midrange is ideal).
When levels are elevated, it means the person is not digesting fats, proteins, or carbohydrates well. This is maldigestion and malabsorption. In short, they will not get the nutrients needed to power up the body.

Calprotectin, EPX, Lactoferrin, and Lysozyme. Inflammation markers (in the green zone).
If in the yellow or red zone, a specific supplement will be needed.

Note: Discover what bothers the gut and get rid of it. Is it offending foods, stress/cortisol issues, NSAIDS, ETOH, BCPs, antacids/acid-blocking medication (such as PPIs for example), metformin, etc.?

Note: Elevation of calprotectin, lactoferrin, and/or lysozyme indicates not only inflammation, but also that the patient is advancing toward colon cancer, ulcerative colitis, and Crohn's disease.[92] If this number is not back to a normal reference range by the first recheck, **the patient should be referred for colonoscopy**.

Note: An elevated EPX often means some foods have a negative impact on the gut.[93,94]

Sig A (midrange)
High Sig A means intestinal permeability issues, better known as a 'leaky gut.' With a low Sig A, the person has lost the protective

mucosal membrane separating the intestinal wall from the contents of the gut.[93,94]

N-butyrate and the SCFAs (short-chain fatty acids) (high end of the range)
When N-butyrate is low, so much inflammation is produced, the individual has an increased risk of colon cancer.[93,94] The good bacteria in the gut should make these crucial SCFAs, and butter is the sole food source of butyrate.

Beta Glucuronidase (midrange)
Low beta-glucuronidase levels indicate tolerance issues with carbohydrates, including blood sugar.[93,94] High levels of Beta glucuronidase indicate toxicity and also raise the risk of colon cancer.[93,94] Also, when this marker is high, estrogens that should be expelled are reactivated and reabsorbed into the body, further contributing to estrogen dominance.[93,94] The same goes for all other toxins. "The good bacteria should make an enzyme to break down beta-glucuronidase to keep levels optimal."[32]

Good and Bad Microbes (high in the good and low/none of the bad)
The status of the intestinal microbiome is imperative. This refers to the balance of the good and bad microorganisms that populate our gut. Lab companies are starting to incorporate specific reports about the overall diversity these days. However, the abundance of some of the most important individual organisms is also reported. At present, these involve 3-6 specific ones. Levels go from no growth (NG) to 4+, the ideal range.

"Bad" bacterial numbers are reported as well. Some "bad" bacteria are only really "bad" when they reach levels of 4+. Others are bad enough to require attention when they are at 1+. "Mold is similar to bad bacteria, but tends to be hard to find and diagnose."[32]

A popular digestive stool analysis company (Doctor's Data) looks for microscopic mold spores; this test helps to identify the presence of problematic amounts of mold. Mold infections are problematic and can be difficult to clear.

PROVOCATIVE HEAVY METAL: INTERPRETATION
(See Figure 10)

In figure 10, notice heavy metal levels both within and outside of the reference range.

Toxic Metals; Urine

TOXIC METALS		RESULTS µg/g creat	REFERENCE INTERVAL		WITHIN REFERENCE	OUTSIDE REFERENCE
Aluminum	(Al)	1.9	<	35		
Antimony	(Sb)	0.7	<	0.2		
Arsenic	(As)	11	<	80		
Barium	(Ba)	2	<	7		
Beryllium	(Be)	< dl	<	1		
Bismuth	(Bi)	< dl	<	4		
Cadmium	(Cd)	0.7	<	1		
Cesium	(Cs)	11	<	10		
Gadolinium	(Gd)	0.1	<	0.8		
Lead	(Pb)	13	<	2		
Mercury	(Hg)	1.7	<	4		
Nickel	(Ni)	2	<	10		
Palladium	(Pd)	< dl	<	0.15		
Platinum	(Pt)	< dl	<	0.1		
Tellurium	(Te)	< dl	<	0.5		
Thallium	(Tl)	0.5	<	0.5		
Thorium	(Th)	< dl	<	0.03		
Tin	(Sn)	0.8	<	5		
Tungsten	(W)	0.04	<	0.4		
Uranium	(U)	< dl	<	0.04		

URINE CREATININE	RESULTS mg/dL	REFERENCE INTERVAL		-2SD	-1SD	MEAN	+1SD	+2SD
Creatinine	68.3	30 -	225			•		

Figure 10

Note: Some environmental toxins are so harmful even small amounts can lead to significant health problems. Lead is one of those dangerous toxins—and mercury, cadmium, nickel, arsenic, cesium—

to name a few. When the central mechanisms are off, the ability to detoxify suffers along with many other essential bodily functions. Not enough B vitamins to run detoxification pathways, inability to activate/methylate the B vitamins, lack of optimal liver function, etc. Further, "Lack of glutathione to keep mitochondria clear of toxins and making ATP and lack of gut function."[32]

Attempting to avoid environmental toxins isn't as pertinent as removing them quickly. Environmental toxins are everywhere—and it so often starts in the womb, so they can be tough to avoid.

Note: A provocative heavy metal test uses an oral chelating agent to mobilize toxins from fat stores to show up in a urine test. A non-provocative test looks at levels in the urine without a chelating agent. A non-provocative HM test may not be helpful. Often, not enough heavy metals in the liquids of our body (blood and urine) are present at any one time to find the toxins on a non-provocative HM test.

Remember, most toxins that concern us are fat-soluble, not water-soluble. Also, lead and mercury aren't typically excreted through the kidneys: they need to be bound by the chelating agent and "dragged" out of the body via the kidneys.[95]

FOOD SENSITIVITY TEST: INTERPRETATION
(See Figure 11)

The food sensitivity test that I often run assesses about 90 foods for an IgG reaction, a delayed hypersensitivity response. Each food is graded 0-4. The foods of concern, which should be eliminated, are the ones graded 1-4. Zeros are zeros. Often, problematic foods must be excluded for at least four to six weeks, since the half-life of IgG is 21 days.

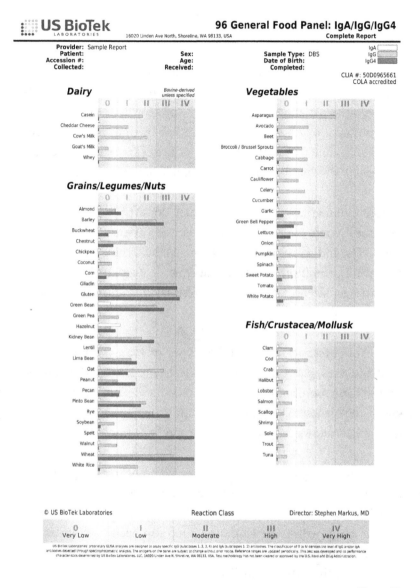

Figure 11

Note: There is a long battle ahead when the gut is so disrupted that certain foods become the body's enemy. In these cases, eliminating the food for a while is not enough. Unlike the 4-6 weeks, it takes longer, because the gut needs to heal first, which always takes more time.

One example is celiac disease, an AD that attacks the small intestine, producing abdominal pain and other gut symptoms, but also diffuse systemic dysfunction.[18,19] All sorts of systemic symptoms with minimal or no gut complaints occur in eight out of 10 celiac patients. It's one reason that four out of five celiac patients are never diagnosed[19,20]—but it's also a great example of the gut's significance.

Simply eliminating gluten from a diet doesn't allow the gut and immune system to reset: celiac disease patients often develop new ADs and chronic diseases in general. These include Type 1 diabetes, multiple sclerosis, anemia, osteoporosis, infertility, miscarriage, seizures, migraines, intestinal cancers, and dermatitis herpetiformis.[18,19]

Note: Some tests can look at 500 types of food products, spices, food additives, etc. I don't use these tests any longer. They provide great information but the body is so good at healing, as long as we know "the biggest fish to fry". Eliminating the most significant foods temporarily allows the body to be in a good position to reset the rest.

When addressing central mechanisms, we want to put the body in a position to start repairing problems on its own. The body is an amazing machine and, most of the time, people can self-correct most of their issues with some guidance. They also need to eliminate any foods that produce an immediate hypersensitivity reaction as well as other toxins from their daily lives.

TREATMENT OPTIONS BASED ON INITIAL LAB DATA

Many of life's failures are people who did not realize how close they were to success when they gave up.

—Thomas Edison

Look at the big picture when making decisions on treatment options—the biggest fish to fry. It's easy to get caught up in the minutia. Patients do it all the time. They may ask: "I was reading about a supplement for this symptom, should I start using it?" Keep in mind, while treating people with complex multiorgan system dysfunction, we need to address the central mechanisms; not chase individual symptoms with specific supplements or medications.

By addressing the central mechanisms, the patient can fix all their issues at the same time. As time goes on and some symptoms change quicker than others, now give special attention to slower to change symptoms. What I tell patients is, less is more, "If a particular symptom clears as we address the central mechanisms, we will be happy we didn't waste your time and money using a supplement for just that issue. Your body was able to fix that on its own. If it's slow to change compared with other improvements, we can give it special attention so it improves like the other areas."

INITIAL RECOMMENDATIONS FOR EVERYONE

- Always address cortisol in anyone in their mid-teens or older. Start an adrenal adaptogen, and make sure they do daily relaxation exercises. On occasion, L-theanine may be substituted for the adrenal adaptogen.
- Start DHEA if blood and/or saliva results are lower than ideal.
- Start Vitamin D restoration.
- Start treating chronic infections.
- Perform a food sensitivity test (FST) if the patient was asked to avoid wheat/gluten and cow's milk dairy on the initial visit but didn't see significant improvement in their multiorgan system problems. Remember, the elimination diet can be used if the patient is unable to do the FST.
- Start a probiotic if a patient is not already on one.
- Consider starting a high-quality multivitamin (as opposed to several individual nutrient supplements) if a person is low on most or all of the nutrients tested.

BLOOD WORK: TREATMENT

RBC Magnesium
Magnesium glycinate: Preferred if muscle involvement is not a primary component of the symptoms, but there are other symptoms of magnesium deficiency such as anxiety, insomnia, constipation, and blood sugar issues.[96]

Dosage: Magnesium Glycinate 1-2, twice per day (Douglas Laboratories)

Magnesium Malate
Use this form of magnesium if muscle involvement is a primary component of the patient's symptoms.

Dosage: Magnesium Malate 1-2, twice per day (Douglas Laboratories).

Note: The dose of both forms of magnesium can go higher to reach the desired therapeutic effect. Decrease dose if diarrhea occurs.

Note: A magnesium workaround. Consider having a patient use Epsom salt baths (magnesium sulfate) three or more evenings a week rather than oral magnesium supplementation. This can be a less expensive option as well as a more effective way of getting magnesium into the body. Remember, the gut is disrupted and not digesting and absorbing nutrients. Absorption through the skin may be much easier. The warm water and the magnesium salts in a bath near bedtime can help the individual get a better night's sleep as well.

RBC Zinc Low
Tissue cannot heal without zinc.[97]

Dosage: Zn-Zyme Forte 1-2, twice per day (Biotics Research).

Ferritin High
Have the patient donate blood 1-2 times, 4-6 weeks apart.

Ferritin Low
Dosage: HemePlex Fe, 1-2 capsules, twice per day, or higher as tolerated (NuMedica).

CoQ 10 Low
Dosage: CoQ-Clear 100, 2 capsules daily with food (NuMedica). Can go up to 3-4 daily or more.

Homocysteine High
Dosage: Methyl-Plex B, 1 capsule twice per day (NuMedica).

L-glutamine

Note: Consider immediately adding the amino acid L-glutamine in a powdered form if neuropathic pain is a primary complaint, or if the neurogenic symptoms are slow to change.

Dosage: L-Glutamine powder, 3-5 grams, 2-3 times a day (NuMedica). Between meals on an empty stomach for gut and systemic symptoms. Okay to take with food if only used for systemic symptoms.

Note: L-glutamine can convert to glutamate. Excessive glutamate can be problematic for the brain. Although this would suggest starting slow with L-glutamine in situations involving brain issues this tends not to be the case. Starting at the usual doses tends to be well tolerated and can help with brain-related issues. Helping the gut helps the brain in addition to L-glutamine's ability to repair the nervous system as a whole. Not just the peripheral nervous system as mentioned above, but the central nervous system as well.

Vitamin B-12 Low

Dosage: Methyl-B12 Rx, 1 sublingual daily (NuMedica). Can increase to 2-3 sublinguals daily as needed.

Note: Oftentimes there is no need to use a specific B12 product as the amount of B12 available in high quality, fully activated, fully methylated B complex will be enough. Such as with the Methyl Plex B from NuMedica. When patients present with chronic central and peripheral nervous system issues (including anxiety, depression, panic attacks, bipolar disorder, etc.), additional B12 may be needed. Even though everyone should have a B12 level of $\geq$ 800-900, some people need to be a lot higher to achieve optimal benefit.

Vitamin D

Dosage: D3-5000, 1-3 capsules daily with food (NuMedica).

Note: If vitamin D levels on testing are out-of-the-range low and the person is quite sick, consider 5-10 caps daily for 5-7 days, then decrease to the standard dose.

Thyroid
Dosage: T4 thyroid medication (examples include Synthroid and Levothyroxine), 25-50mcg, take in the morning on an empty stomach. Increase dose as needed following subsequent testing.

Dosage: Desiccated thyroid (example Armour Thyroid), 30-60mg daily empty stomach.

Important Note: Cortisol issues should be treated for at least one month before there will be any noticeable differences with thyroid treatment. That being said, taking care of the cortisol issues and addressing vitamin and mineral deficiencies will help the body detoxify better with B-vitamins and gut restoration. The individual may already be a better thyroid converter and no change to the T4 medication needs to be made after working through the cortisol issues. If thyroid medication is started before a month has been spent addressing cortisol, the patient may feel no better or even feel worse—even if appropriate medication and a suitable initial dose was used.

DHEA
Dosage (women): 25-50 mg (NuMedica) taken in the morning on an empty stomach. In women without an AD, start with 5-10mg taken in the morning on an empty stomach.

Dosage (men): 25-50 mg (NuMedica) taken in the morning on an empty stomach.

Note: With hormone restoration, always "start low and go slow." Always start with a dose on the lower end of the treatment range.

Note: I often have patients take DHEA at the same time as their thyroid medicines (taken in the morning on an empty stomach) rather than taking thyroid medication 45-60 minutes before breakfast and the DHEA 1-2 hours after breakfast. When the doses are split over time, it's easier for patients to forget their DHEA.

Note: DHEA (NuMedica): You can use 5mg or 25mg capsules.

Celiac Disease
Dosage: Wheat Rescue 1 capsule before a meal (Microbiome Labs).

Note: It can be difficult to completely eliminate gluten. Hidden gluten can be found in modified food starches, preservatives and food stabilizers, prescription and over-the-counter medications, vitamins and mineral supplements, herbal and nutritional supplements, lipstick, toothpaste and mouthwash, envelope and stamp glue, and even in Play-Dough.[98]

Note: Use Wheat Rescue if the person doesn't have complete oversight of the foods they eat. It should be used for any patient with celiac disease. For AD patients in general, it can also protect them from the effects of wheat contamination when eating outside their homes.

pH Structured Silver Solution
Dosing often starts at 4 ounces once a day (swish for 1-2 minutes and swallow) for 4 days; then, 2 ounces a day.

Dosage (adults): 4 oz daily for 4 days then 2oz per day.
Dosage (children): 1 tsp, twice a day.

Biocidin LSF and Biocidin
Dosage: Biocidin LSF (liposomal biocidin) and Biocidin (Advanced Liquid Biocidin): For the dosage chart for adults and children visit *www.DrDavidBilstrom.com/npadguide.*

SPECIAL SECTION: SEX HORMONE RESTORATION

Optimal estrogen and testosterone restoration without creating new issues is an advanced strategy of hormone restoration. Many practitioners use estrogen and testosterone therapy, but few do it well, or even safely. They're not:

- Appropriately testing either before or during treatment.
- Monitoring the excessive conversion of estradiol (good estrogen) to estrone (not-so-good estrogen).
- Monitoring estradiol levels well enough to know when the patient is overtreated.
- Testing for the excessive conversion of testosterone to DHT (dihydrotestosterone).
- Using progesterone with estrogens or estrogens with testosterone in female patients.

Given that all hormones are great anti-inflammatory agents, restoring hormone status is vital. However, doing it correctly is even more important. Doing nothing is better than creating new problems.

A special way to optimize hormones without using estrogens, progesterone, and testosterone is to use the steroidogenic hormone production cascade. (Thank you, Dr. Mark L. Gordon).

The body is so elegant in its methods. Letting the body heal itself is one of the most important concepts. This applies to hormone restoration as well—having the hormones available and in optimal balance. Remember, when it comes to hormones, the entire "symphony orchestra" has to be well-balanced. Thus, let's become familiar with the steroidogenic hormone production cascade.

To begin, cholesterol is the 'mother of all hormones' in women, and the 'father of all hormones' in men. LDL cholesterol, to be precise. The liver makes LDL cholesterol. With elevated levels of LDL on blood testing and total cholesterol (TC) appearing as elevated LDL, we must ask ourselves, "Why would the liver make more cholesterol than seems appropriate?" A good reason is that the body is self-correcting. It is feeding the steroidogenic hormone production cascade to optimize hormone status. Giving patients medicine to lower cholesterol levels in this situation guarantees the body will not reestablish a suitable hormone balance: chronic disease just keeps rolling along.

The old way of thinking was "we get old so we stop making hormones." However, the truth is the complete opposite, "we stop making hormones so we get old." We start breaking down, getting old, unable to keep the body healthy and happy like it should be at least until we are 90.

When cortisol levels are stuck in the 'on' position, cholesterol gets shunted toward cortisol production. This leaves too little cholesterol to make all the other hormones within the steroidogenic hormone production cascade.

I like to explain it to patients this way. "If you have four children, and one requires so much of your time, the others don't get the attention they deserve." Almost every adult will understand this concept. All my patients nod their heads in agreement.

The first hormone to become depleted in this situation tends to be progesterone. Thus, estrogen dominance begins, and the eventual development of AD starts in earnest. Because progesterone is one of the few calming hormones, cortisol is in trouble when it loses its good friend progesterone.

Let me tell you a beautiful workaround when it comes to correcting the steroidogenic hormone production cascade. And I must thank Dr. Mark L. Gordon and his book, *The Clinical Application of Interventional Endocrinology* for this one. Rather than giving patients the 'downstream hormones' estrogen and testosterone and worrying about under or over-treating; watching excessive conversion to undesirable hormones; about which form of estrogen or testosterone to use—the body does that work itself. We can let the body figure out how much of the downstream hormones it needs by giving it some of the upstream hormones — at least until it can create the upstream hormones on its own.

This involves starting the patient on DHEA and pregnenolone, feeding the steroidogenic hormone production cascade. The pregnenolone will convert to progesterone. The DHEA will transform into testosterone and estrogen.

In due course, as the cortisol stuck in the "fight or flight" mode is corrected (partially because absent/unbalanced hormones are not causing physical stress to the system 24 hours a day), cholesterol will become available to make the other essential hormones. The body itself will produce DHEA, pregnenolone, progesterone, estradiol, estrone, testosterone. The liver will no longer need to make high levels of LDL cholesterol and lipid levels will normalize. The body is so elegant in its ability to self-correct and maintain health. Or return to health, as the case may be.

Sex Hormone Restoration (Steroidogenic Hormone Production Cascade)

Dosage: DHEA at the dosages often used (NuMedica) along with pregnenolone at common doses (NuMedica). Increasing the doses as needed, based on hormone levels when retested.

Note: It is vital to create calm in the body and begin to address estrogen dominance early on: starting a patient on progesterone right away is often a great idea. In time, decrease progesterone dosage or stop it altogether, once production of the steroidogenic hormone production cascade has been reestablished.

Downstream Hormones

Estrogens
Dosage: Compounded BiEst 80/20 cream. Reasonable starting dose 1mg/ml, ½-1ml in the morning. This dose can be increased slowly, ½-1mg at a time, to a max of 3-5mg/ml, ½-1ml over time.

Note: Avoid a cream that is either too concentrated or too diluted. If it is too concentrated, absorption will be compromised. If too diluted, there will be so much cream spread on the skin, it will get messy and absorption will also be compromised.

Note: This is imperative, I need to emphasize it a second time. A woman should <u>never</u> take estrogen without also being on progesterone, even if they no longer have a uterus. They work hand in hand: progesterone makes strong bones and estrogen prevents excessive bone loss. Estrogen can irritate breast tissue and progesterone protects breast tissue.

Note: Only use bio-identical hormones.

Progesterone
Dosage, oral (prescription): 100mg either 1-2 hours before bedtime, if falling asleep is part of insomnia. Use at bedtime if staying asleep is an issue, but falling asleep is not a problem.

Note: I almost always use progesterone orally for all the reasons outlined in the lab interpretation section.

Dosage, topical (compounded prescription): 10-20mg/ml at ½-1ml q.p.m.

Note: Progesterone has been available orally and topically. More recently it is also available as an implanted pellet. All routes of administration "may work equally well, except oral progesterone tends to be much better at controlling insomnia and anxiety."[32] The benefit of oral progesterone may also be seen much sooner than that of topical progesterone—often as fast as two to five days. Thus, doses can be rapidly raised for optimal correction of estrogen dominance and other issues. Just as with topical bioidentical estrogens, if topical progesterone is used, it might take four to eight weeks to start to see the effect.

When using oral bioidentical progesterone, a reasonable starting dose for most women will be 100mg. This is the lowest prescription dose available at a typical non-compounding pharmacy. If dosing is at bedtime but a woman feels groggy the next morning, then move the dosing to 1-2 hours before bedtime again. Feeling groggy the next day suggests the person is a poor detoxifier and has problems clearing the medicine from their systems. And will also have trouble clearing anything else from the system.

Sometimes, 100 mg is more than a woman needs. Using a compounding pharmacy for a 25 mg capsule, increasing by 25 mg every two to five days until optimal symptom control is achieved, is a good option.

Note: "Pulsing of hormone restoration is vital. A woman's body likes to see different amounts of sex hormones on different days.

In premenopausal women, topical/oral progesterone use will be cycled."[32]

Premenopausal women will seldom need extra estrogen. Progesterone is used on days 14-25 of the cycle and avoided on days 26-30. If symptoms return to an unacceptable extent on the off days, progesterone can be restarted, but at perhaps half the usual dose. Initially, though, a woman may need the same therapeutic dose of progesterone every night of the month. They may just not feel as well on the nights when a lower dose, or none, is taken. As they improve, the pulsing of hormones will be better tolerated.

Note: "In perimenopausal and postmenopausal women, a pulsing schedule of the BiEst and progesterone might be Monday through Saturday, and off Sunday."[32]

Testosterone
Dosage for women (topical only): Topical compounded 0.5 mg/ml at ½-1ml daily to start.

Dosage for men (topical only): compounded topical 10-20 mg/ml at ½-1ml daily to start.

Dosage for men (IM): 50-100 mg IM q week to start. Dosage may eventually need to be 150-200 mg IM weekly.

Note: When using testosterone in men and women topically, watch for excessive conversion to DHT (Dihydrotestosterone). Decrease the dose if this happens.

Note: When using IM testosterone in men, watch for excessive conversion to estradiol and estrone. Decrease the dose if this happens.

SALIVA CORTISOL: TREATMENT

No matter what state of disruption cortisol is in and no matter what causes the disruption, calm needs to be created. Along with addressing all drivers of AD, including the physical and biochemical stressors, a person needs to reestablish the "relaxation mode." Free apps are available, such as "Insight Timer" and "Calm." Alternatively, use Nature. Or music therapy. There are so many options to help the body reestablish calm. For more information visit *www.DrDavidBilstrom. com/npadguide.*

For anyone older than their mid-teens, a supplement called an adrenal adaptogen will be vital to reset cortisol and allow the body to heal. This supplement is filled with herbs and vitamins that help the adrenal gland feel a sense of calm.[99] It is difficult for the body to heal when it is in perpetual stress mode. At ages younger than mid-teens, the body is so fantastic at healing. Fixing the biochemical stressors and doing relaxation exercises such as the ones mentioned above, is usually adequate for them. They don't tend to need adrenal adaptogen supplements. Since it is an "adaptogen", it is balancing, not directional. It does not push the cortisol up or down. It just allows the body/cortisol to go the way it should to heal. If someone is low they will come up. If they are high, they will come down. If a person has a combination of high and low, all cortisol levels will move toward the ideal state. Of course, the biochemical stressors must also be addressed to give the cortisol a chance to reset. Many folks have come to me having done regular relaxation activities for a very long time and still don't feel as well as they had hoped. This is because a person will never "relax" their way out of an AD if they still consume foods that bother them, or they have a fungal infection of the gut, etc.

Dosage: AdrenaMed, 1 capsule two times a day (NuMedica). Take it with breakfast and lunch.

Note: If taken late in the day, the patient may experience insomnia.

DIGESTIVE STOOL ANALYSIS: TREATMENT

A couple of testing companies do digestive stool analysis. Some practitioners prefer one over the other, I prefer to use both. Some insurance companies work better with a particular testing company. Testing will identify the most important issues to treat. The body will often take care of the rest of the problems.

Pancreatic elastase (enzymes) If <500, start digestive enzymes or apple cider vinegar (ACV) before meals. Both help the patient digest their food better but the ACV also heals the gut.

Dosage enzymes: Pan-V, 1-2 caps before meals (NuMedica).

Dosage ACV: 2 tsp (mixed in water) before meals (Bragg's with "the mother." Available at most grocery stores).

Protein Products and Fecal Fat
If high, then a person is not digesting fats and/or proteins well.

Dosage: Start with Pan-V (NuMedica) or the ACV. See dosages above.

Calprotectin, Lysozyme, Lactoferrin, and EPX.
Depending on which company runs the stool analysis, different inflammation markers will be tested. If high, then excessive inflammation is present.

Dosage: L-glutamine powder, 3-5mgs, 2-3 times a day on an empty stomach (NuMedica).

Note: It is of great concern if calprotectin, lactoferrin, or lysozyme are elevated. At this point, the individual is moving toward diseases such as ulcerative colitis, Crohn's disease, and colon cancer.[92]

Treating what is found in all the testing, not just the stool analysis, will start to eliminate this inflammation."[32] To clear this issue quickly—L-glutamine powder must be included.

Note: If the retesting three months after starting treatment is not in the ideal range, the person should have a colonoscopy.

EPX
"When this is high, it suggests food is bothering the gut."[32] Avoiding the offending foods should drop this number by the next retest. If it's still high, the patient either needs to better avoid foods already identified, or additional foods may be problematic and should be eliminated from the diet. "Sometimes, empirically, some foods may need to be removed for a while."[32] For example, lectin-containing foods or the nightshades, including legumes, tomatoes, potatoes, eggplant.

Sig A (secretory IgA): treat whether too high or too low.
Dosage: L-glutamine 3-5gms, 2-3 times a day on an empty stomach.

Note: Also, think of Sig A as an inflammation marker. If it's too high, there might be the presence of an intestinal permeability disorder. "If too low, it suggests the patient has also lost the protective membrane that separates the gut wall from the gut contents."[32]

Note: When it comes to Sig A restoration, start to think now about the findings you will see on retesting. If a low result got high at the time of a retest, that is good news. "The protective membrane has been reestablished, but the intestinal permeability disorder still needs to be corrected."[32] If the patient is high at first, but is found to be low on retesting, then a loss of the protective mucosal membrane has been added to the original leaky gut.

N-Butyrate
Dosage: Butyric Cal-Mag, 1-2, twice per day (NuMedica).

Note: N-butyrate and the other SCFAs in a healthy gut, should be produced in adequate amounts by the good bacteria. When you observe low levels on the first digestive stool analysis results sheet, you may wish to wait and see if it self-corrects with the other interventions. If it still is not optimal by retest, treat it with the Butyric Cal-Mag.

Beta Glucuronidase
Dosage: Calcium D-glucarate, 1-2 capsules, twice per day (NuMedica).

Note: The excessive level of beta-glucuronidase will tend to self-correct as the gut heals. The good bacteria should make an enzyme to break down the beta-glucuronidase and prevent the accumulation of excessive amounts. If this does not improve by the second stool test, consider calcium D-glucarate supplementation. Or, if the level is extreme and you suspect toxicity is a big issue (including the reactivation and reabsorption of old, toxic estrogens creating estrogen dominance), start this supplement right away.

Note: Another option would be to use a supplement like Fiber Factors (NuMedica). This is a combination supplement made up of soluble and insoluble fiber. The soluble fiber helps to feed the good bacteria in the gut. The insoluble fiber will bind up toxins and will keep them from being reabsorbed back into the bloodstream. Instead, they end up in the toilet where they belong.

Dosage: Fiber Factors 1 dose 1-2 times a day (NuMedica).

Good Bacteria
Dosage: Megasporebiotic, 2 capsules daily with food (Microbiome Labs).

Dosage: HiFlora-50$_{12}$, 2 capsules daily (NuMedica).

Note: My preference is to start with Megaspore, then alternate with the HiFlora-50$_{12}$ every three months.

Note: High-quality probiotics and Vitamin D will always be required.

Infections: Bacterial
Dosage: pH Structured Silver Solution, at 4 ozs/day for four days; then, 2 oz/day. Use for six weeks. Wait four weeks after stopping and retest digestive stool analysis. This nanosilver has an easier dosing schedule (once a day) than Biocidin. Thus, my first choice is pH Structured Silver Solution.

Dosage: Advanced Liquid Biocidin: See specific dosing schedule instruction sheet (Bio-Botanical Research) or go to *www. DrDavidBilstrom.com/npadguide*. Use for six weeks. Wait four weeks and retest digestive stool analysis.

Note: Consider using GI Detox (Bio-Botanical Research) along with the Advanced Liquid Biocidin. For a dosing schedule see *www. DrDavidBilstrom.com/npadguide*.

Note: Antibiotics will be problematic for the gut and immune system. Thus, whenever an antibiotic is used, each dose should be followed 2 hours later by a probiotic. The probiotic should be continued daily for 2 weeks after completing the course of antibiotics. But when looking at taking antibiotics for an entire month to have a chance to clear a gut bacterial infection identified on digestive stool analysis, the use of either pH Structured Silver Solution or Biocidin are better options to clear the bad bug without hurting the good bugs.

Infections: Fungal

Dosage: Nystatin, 1,000,000 Units, twice per day, for three months. Wait four weeks and then retest digestive stool analysis.

Note: Fungal infections found on yeast cultures or microscopic yeast (only performed on Doctor's Data digestive stool analysis) reported as "few" or worse, can be stubborn to clear. It will often take three months of using an antimicrobial or a specific antifungal agent.

Note: My recommendation is to use grapefruit seed extract (GFSE) (Pure Encapsulations) for six weeks, in addition to Nystatin. Do not take longer than six weeks, as the GFSE can harm the good bacteria in ways similar to antibiotics. GFSE can be used when there are both fungal and bacterial infections identified on testing. Watch the sensitivity panels on the Doctor's Data digestive stool analysis, to confirm this is a reasonable option for the particular bacterial infection.

Dosage: Grapefruit Seed Extract, one capsule twice per day, for six weeks (Pure Encapsulations).

Importance of Optimizing Vitamin D Receptor (VDR) Sensitivity

It is vital to understand not only vitamin D but also vitamin D receptors (VDRs). Having sensitive vitamin D receptors in the gut (as opposed to vitamin D receptor resistance), along with vitamin D is important for not only gut health but the entire body. This will impact the intestinal microbiome as well as inflammation control systemically and health overall.

An important reason why we know vitamin D is critical for gut health is the sheer number of VDRs present even compared to other tissues. This tells us how important Vitamin D is for the gut. The VDRs need vitamin D on a daily basis to do the essential work needed by the gut and the body as a whole.

Let's review two critical components required for optimal gut and body health—vitamin D and vitamin D receptors (VDRs). The intestinal mucosa contains many vitamin D receptors, making it so important for the gut.[51] VDRs need vitamin D available in the gut to do essential work and maintain good bodily health. However, VDRs need Vitamin D and good bacteria to create optimal amounts of n-butyrate and function properly. All the vitamin D in the world coming into the gut through oral supplementation may not help if we have down-regulated vitamin D receptor sensitivity. This is when the triad of oral, daily, vitamin D optimization, daily probiotics, and n-butyrate supplementation are a great option designed to reestablish the intestinal microbiome and clear excessive inflammation in the gut. Thus, the body has a chance to clear even inflammatory bowel disease, as well as celiac disease flairs. This triad will also help clear the excessive inflammation in the body as a whole, thus addressing chronic disease processes in general.[51]

Dosage: Vitamin D. Daily D3 5000, at the dose identified based on blood work results (NuMedica).

Dosage: Probiotic. Megasporebiotic, 2 daily with food (Microbiome Labs). Or, HiFlora-50$_{12}$ 2 per day (NuMedica).

Dosage: Butyrate. Butyric Cal-Mag, 1-2, twice per day (Biotics Research).

Note: This triad of interventions is powerful at correcting what is wrong with the body. For more information, read the scientific journal article, "Ancient nuclear receptor VDR with new functions: microbiome and inflammation." *Inflammatory Bowel Disease*, May 2018.[51]

GI Panel Infection
Dosage: Use the antimicrobial options as above for any identified infections.

Note: If the antimicrobials we've discussed to clear infections found in the GI Panel are too innovative, use a more standard treatment approach that includes antibiotics. Probiotics taken two hours after each antibiotic dose is essential. This will minimize the negative impact on the good bacteria (including in the gut) while offending infections are cleared.

PROVOCATIVE HEAVY METAL TEST: TREATMENT

Heavy Metals in the Yellow or Red Zones

Dosage: HM Protect, 4 capsules daily for three days and then off for seven days (NuMedica). Repeat for 4-6 months, then retest.

Dosage: Mineral-Plex (NuMedica), 2 capsules, twice per day, on the seven days when—HM Protect is not taken.

Note: HM Protect removes "heavy metals" from the body. But it also clears "good metals" such as magnesium, iron, and zinc, etc. Using Mineral-Plex helps prevent the depletion of the "good metals".

Note: Some people may feel sick on the days of detoxification. This is because they are so full of toxins, to begin with, and/or they have difficulty clearing the toxins once they are mobilized. If this occurs, decrease the number of capsules of HM Protect on the "on" days. Or maybe use them for two days instead of three. Or perhaps, add GI Detox (NuMedica), a combination clay, and charcoal mix, to bind the toxins as they are mobilized so they do not make the individual unwell as the detoxification process occurs.

Note: Consider adding a high-quality fiber supplement (Numedica's Fiber Factors, 1 dose, 1-2 times a day), to bind the toxins after they are dumped into the gut—protecting the body until they can be cleared.

Note: An individual must have at least one bowel movement daily before starting formal detoxification. "If bowel movements are occurring less often, the mobilized toxins will be dumped into the gut, then reabsorbed back into the system."[32] Increasing water intake can be helpful. Take half the person's body weight in pounds, and have them drink that number in ounces of water daily (for a 150 lb person, 150/2=75 ounces of water). Also, consider adding Fiber Factors, 1 dose, 1-2 times a day (NuMedica).

FOOD SENSITIVITY TEST: TREATMENT

An important concept when it comes to AD is that everyone (no exceptions), has a delayed hypersensitivity reaction to the proteins in wheat and cow's milk dairy. An IgG reaction. 62 proteins in wheat bother these individuals and gluten is just one of them. (At least until they have a chance to reset and clear the hypersensitivity reaction to the cow's milk dairy proteins.)

When a person with an AD first presents, if they have never gone wheat/gluten and cow's milk dairy-free for at least 4-6 weeks, I might ask them to do this first before doing a food sensitivity test. In their follow-up visit in 6-8 weeks, if they have avoided these problematic proteins well, they might say, "I can't believe how much better I feel already. This is great." If this is the case, these might be the only two types of proteins bothering them. They may not need a formal food sensitivity test after all. However, if they don't feel a lot better, then a food sensitivity test should be run. Or, at least a food elimination diet should be initiated if they are unable to afford the food sensitivity test.

After the multi-organ system issues have improved a great deal, a good possibility is that they've reset their food sensitivities. Now, formal food challenges can begin.

In a formal food challenge, the patient consumes the food to be tested twice a day, for three days in a row, then pauses for the rest of the week. If everything feels fine, they have reset the food and can eat it again.

If they feel unwell in any way, they have not reset the food yet and should still avoid it. They can re-test every 3-6 months as often as they want, in the hope of eventually resetting the food. It may take several challenges or, despite their best efforts, they may never become tolerant of certain foods. At this point, we are testing delayed hypersensitivity reactions and checking one food at a time. Often, people feel unwell if they haven't reset a certain food by day one, two, or three. But oftentimes it doesn't affect them until days 4-7.

Note: A person should keep a diary of the date and the food being tested, as well as any reactions they experience.

AD patients will never fully reset wheat/gluten proteins. These should be avoided to maintain optimal control over the immune system and avoid the return of dysregulation. "The body actually attacking itself is like going off a cliff: you'll never fully recover."[32] Over time, however, many people will lose much of their sensitivity and can cheat three or four times a year, experiencing mild symptoms of intolerance, rather than the severe reactions they may have experienced before. WheatRescue (Microbiome Labs) at one capsule before a meal can be taken to minimize negative impacts when someone may consume these types of foods.

WHEN AND WHAT TO RETEST

Spread love everywhere you go. Let no one come to you without leaving happier.

—Mother Teresa

It works well to wait three months before retesting, then follow up with the patient when the results are available. The body needs time to make changes. However, with the bloodwork, we might want to retest sooner. Or, for someone with a fungal infection of the gut, treating it with Nystatin for three months (and possibly GFSE for six weeks,) and then retest at the four-month mark is recommended.

BLOOD WORK

I recheck blood work three months later, along with the saliva cortisol and the digestive stool analysis. If the saliva and stool testing results are looking a lot better the second time around, you can choose to wait six months or longer before retesting again. Retesting blood work earlier may need to happen for specific reasons:

- Vitamins and minerals: Often, eight weeks is all that is needed before retesting to see if the changes have worked and if the patient feels better.
- Vitamin D: 4-6 weeks is sufficient to retest after making a dose change.

- Thyroid: If modifying the dose of a T4 thyroid medicine (such as Levothyroxine and Synthroid), wait 6-8 weeks before rechecking levels. If changing the dose of a desiccated thyroid product (such as Armour Thyroid or NP Thyroid), waiting 4-6 weeks will suffice. These time frames are also long enough to see changes in the patient's symptoms that have occurred with the change in the thyroid medication dosages.
- Hormones: Wait the entire three months.
- Infections: I don't typically retest for the infections identified in the original blood work. Once the patient feels 70-80% better at least, I wonder if the chronic, systemic infections identified on initial blood work are gone. I then take the patient off the broad-spectrum antimicrobial supplement and monitor how they feel. Once they still feel great without it—no backsliding in symptom control—the infections have cleared. And (fingers crossed), the immune system dysregulation is so much better, the infections will never find their way back into the patient's body.

If they feel unwell after stopping the antimicrobial agent (usually they know within the first couple of days), restart the antimicrobial. If the supplement is restarted fast enough, they usually feel better again within a few days. Two months after restarting, stop the antimicrobial supplement again. Keep doing this at two-month intervals until the patient can go without it and still feel just as good.

Note: Occasionally, we need to recheck for infections that were positive on the original blood test. I only do this if the patient didn't take the antimicrobial agent as recommended and/or stopped it before they were feeling much better. As they stopped it prematurely, it has been tough to reach the 70-80% overall improvement.

If the antibody titers are not significantly lower on retesting compared with their baseline, I ask them to restart the antimicrobial and take it until they do feel 70-80% better. Then, stop it again. If backsliding occurs, keep doing this at two-month intervals, until the patient can go without and still feel as well.

Celiac testing: If the individual was close to CD level titers on original testing and had difficulty adhering to an almost 100% wheat/gluten-free nutritional plan, I might retest the CD labs—especially if the patient's symptoms are not much better. I do this because they might have transitioned to actual CD, and wheat proteins, including gluten, are now "battery acid bad": not just a sensitivity anymore.

SALIVA CORTISOL

More often than not, you should wait three months to retest. If the person was crashing their cortisol on original testing, make sure you caught the crash, and they're not in a state of hypocortisolism. Once the crash has been prevented, the cortisol results are headed in the right direction, and if they reestablished a good rhythm, saliva cortisol retesting can wait 6-12 months. When they are feeling much better and doing a good job with establishing calm in their bodies, either retest the cortisol or have them pause their adrenal adaptogen (AdrenaMed) or L-theanine (NuMedica). Restart the supplements if they feel worse without them.

DIGESTIVE STOOL TEST

Retest in three months if no infections were found on original testing. If infections were detected, then retesting should occur four weeks after discontinuation of the antimicrobial agent.

PROVOCATIVE HEAVY METAL (HM) TEST

Rechecking 4-6 months after starting formal detoxification is appropriate. At the first retest, we want to see if the detox program is working. The only way we know it's working before the retest is if the patient felt ill on the days when detox supplements were taken. If they feel worse (on their "on" days), we know toxins are being mobilized as they should. At the first retest, we will see if our efforts are paying off.

But don't expect to complete the detox efforts after 4-6 months. The toxins are difficult to clear. Often it takes 2-4 or more rounds of detox, each 4-6 months long, to rid enough toxins to keep the patient well long-term. By this time, we've repaired their detox pathways, including their gut, to avoid re-accumulation of internal and environmental toxins over time, ever again. We don't need to get their toxic load identified on testing down to zero. The body doesn't need to be perfect, just perfect enough.

Note: This is critical. Get everything into the mid to low green zone in all identified toxins before patients, who want to be parents, conceive. This will help optimize epigenetics, in the parents, prior to conception, and in at least the next four generations. Preventing disease for generations to come!

FOOD SENSITIVITY TEST (FST)

I seldom retest the FST. If someone has avoided the foods identified as problematic, the titers on testing should fall. To retest and find the offending food titers at zero, we can't determine if it's because they are no longer sensitive to it, or if they've just been good at avoiding the food. This is why, when the person feels well enough and has had a good chance of resetting the food, formal food challenges should begin.

The only time I ever recheck the FST is if the patient hasn't been avoiding the offending foods well, or has not improved as much as expected. Or, gut symptoms continue despite all our efforts, perhaps because infections have been so difficult to clear. Retesting will tell us if they've developed new food sensitivities before we could fix their gut. They should still avoid the original offending foods, even if the titers have gone to zero. Once again, only bring these foods back in after successful formal food challenges.

WHEN TO SIMPLIFY AND WHAT TO USE LONG TERM

You have brains in your head. You have feet in your shoes.
You can steer yourself any direction you choose.

—Dr. Seuss

Once the patient returns for follow-up feeling healthier, it's time to consider simplifying the supplement regimen. There is no specific time frame, but if someone is 60-90% better, then it's likely time. They may have already run out of some of the supplements, despite being instructed not to do so.

As the saying goes, "it always takes more to get good, than to stay good." It always takes more supplements, more medication, more relaxation, more time with the counselor, more clean eating to *get* well than it takes to stay well. As you begin to wean down on supplements, keep the person active with lifestyle changes. These self-care skills will help them better tolerate simplifying supplement and medication regimens.

THE SUPPLEMENT REGIMEN

See if the patient can stop a supplement, and still feel well. This means the body has taken over and can take care of itself without the help of the supplement. If a person feels worse after stopping something, their body is saying, "You might feel well enough to think you can stop that supplement. But, I don't agree."

Restart the supplement and try stopping it again in two months. Continue until the person is okay without it. It could be something that they need long-term.

One of the best initial changes is to go from individual vitamin or mineral supplements to a high-quality multivitamin. Perhaps original testing identified deficiencies in some crucial vitamins and minerals, but not all that were tested. So instead of beginning with a multivitamin, you chose a few specific supplements. Now you may suggest, "When you run out, let's stop the Methyl Plex B, the Magnesium Malate, and the Heme Plex Fe. Instead, we'll start a multivitamin with iron. It has some B vitamins, magnesium, and iron, as well as a lot of micronutrients your gut and body need. Your gut needs Vitamin C and Vitamin A found in the multivitamin to heal and stay healthy long term."

Use the same strategy with antimicrobials taken long term to clear chronic infections noted on original blood work. See how they feel without them. If the infections are gone, the person can stop the pH Structured Silver Solution, for example, and feel just as good without it. If not, they will feel worse after a couple of days.

It could take a few weeks to backslide and it may be subtle, so be careful. Often, the backslide will be dramatic. The patient can restart the pH Structured Silver Solution or Biocidin after a few days, and because they were not off it long, they will feel well again after a couple of days.

Note: Despite giving patients this information, I'll get a message a few weeks later, saying they have some new health problems. They may truly be new problems, but they're often old issues returning. To the patient, they may seem new because they were gone for some time before stopping the antimicrobial agents. I ask, "Did these problems begin only after you stopped the pH Structured Silver Solution?" And sure enough, it was. They are instructed to restart the antimicrobial and we plan to try stopping it again in two months.

Ideally, there are only two supplements everyone with an AD needs to take long term. A daily dose of vitamin D, and some probiotics. The gut, and of course the immune system that surrounds the gut, will need them to stay healthy long-term. You may only need the probiotic once or twice a week—not necessarily every day. But, everyone is unique. Some people may feel best long-term if they stay on additional supplements as well. Maybe a multivitamin, for example, because their gut still has difficulty absorbing nutrients. Or, a digestive enzyme. Or, additional magnesium, etc.

Alternating the probiotic used every three months is ideal. My patients often alternate the Megasporebiotic and the HiFlora-50$_{12}$ every three months.

THE MEDICATION REGIMEN

Timing the weaning of medications is similar to that for the supplements. On the original visit, discuss the ultimate goal of weaning down and off most, if not all, their medications. I might say something like, "Once you feel 60-70-80-90% better, we will start to wean down and try to come off some or all of the medicines. Eventually, your body will do the work and you will no longer need so much help from medicines."

It may also be important to share at the first visit, or early on while reversing the autoimmune process, that all medicines have downsides/side effects, even if they provide some benefit.

For example, blood pressure (BP) medicines. If a person has high BP, they don't want to have a stroke. So the medications can put a band-aid on the problem and bring the BP down. You're not actually fixing the reason their BP went up in the first place, but at least they won't have a stroke. This should buy the patient time to figure out why their BP went up, and repair the problem. Their BP starts to come down and they won't need the BP medication anymore.

Why is it important to come off a BP med, if at all possible? They tend to cause vitamin B deficiencies, which cause homocysteine levels to go up. High homocysteine levels increase the chance of the patient having not only a heart attack or stroke but also cancer, Alzheimer's, osteoporosis, mood issues, etc. Yes, the very medicine being used to protect a person from a stroke can eventually increase the risk of a stroke and other bad things, too.

Thus, with medications, use as low a dose as possible, for the shortest duration possible, to get the benefits without the downsides.

Even over-the-counter meds can have awful side effects. We know how bad the NSAIDs are, including gut, kidney, and heart issues. However, acetaminophen also has a significant downside. It depletes the body of the vital substance, glutathione. Glutathione is the most potent free radical scavenger our body makes. Free radical production causes oxidative stress, which creates inflammation, which creates all chronic diseases. It's a terrible idea to deplete glutathione. Even acetaminophen should be avoided, if possible.

Patients are often so tired of the medications by the time they see you, they may start pulling back on their own. They say, "I haven't used Tylenol, Advil, or Percocet since last time." Or, "My blood pressure was getting too low, so I cut the dose in half." If a patient decreases the dose of a medication or stops it altogether, and still feels fine the body is doing the work itself.

IMMUNOSUPPRESSANTS

Let's consider the medicines that have been used specifically for suppressing the immune system. This is an interesting situation. In a perfect world, we'd just send the patient back to the practitioner who is prescribing the medications, and ask them to start to wean the patient down and off the medications as much as able; going as slow or fast as is appropriate for the specific medication.

However, until we have transformed autoimmune disease care worldwide, it will be difficult to get other medical practitioners to help wean patients off these medications. This is one reason why you are so critical in the revolution to reverse and prevent all autoimmunity.

Most medical practitioners are under the impression that patients need to take these prescription medications all their lives. They may say to the patient, either during the original visit when the diagnosis was made or when the patient asks to have the medication weaned down, "There is no way for us to know why you got this AD. There is no way for us to make it go away. You need to be on meds the rest of your life."

What these practitioners are really saying is, "*I do not know* why you got this AD. *I do not know* how to make this AD go away." They don't know, but *now you do!*

Everyone in medicine knows their stuff, but no one knows everything. Don't ask me to prescribe the medicines often used in people with ADs. I have no clue what medications to use, the doses, or what side effects to expect. I don't know how often to check liver function tests when using a certain medication. Or when the side effects of the medication have become so problematic that a new medication needs to be prescribed.

The practitioner who originally wrote the prescription may request the patient not change their medication doses, and to keep taking them forever. That same practitioner could say the same to you, even though you got the patient to the point of potentially not needing the medications any longer.

It can be worth the effort to discuss with the practitioner why your patient, or you, are asking to have the doses weaned down, and ideally, stopped altogether. Explain how the autoimmune process can be reversed by addressing the causes behind the AD, based on specific diagnostic testing. The person is 80-90% better in all areas, not just in the AD symptoms that were still present despite the use of the prescribed medications.

The reality is that often, the decisions of the patients themselves, with your direction, are the only way to do the weaning process. Once we, the experts in reversing and preventing all autoimmunity, have changed the way autoimmune diseases are treated worldwide, it won't be such an issue. It will be common knowledge that this is how it goes with ADs. But for now, it may be left up to you and your patient. Once again, the patient may take the lead. "Usually, I get my infusion every eight weeks and start to feel worse about three weeks before the next infusion. But since I last saw you, I felt great up to the next infusion. So this time, I waited to get the next infusion until I started to feel the symptoms come back and I was able to go fourteen weeks. I want to try and go as long as I can next time as well."

They are already doing what is needed to stop the prescription medications. If they can stay well without them, there's no reason to continue. They may say, "I was feeling so good, I cut my dose of the oral medicine in half six weeks ago, and I am still fine." Or, "I was feeling so good, I tried to decrease my dose by half. But after three weeks I started to feel my symptoms again, so I went back up to my regular dose." That's fine, too. Just like our approach to supplements, we let the body have the final say as to whether it's ready to pull back from the interventions, or not. We are the time-keepers on this journey, waiting a couple of months and ready to try again.

LONG TERM FOLLOW-UP

Only a life lived for others is a life worthwhile.

—Albert Einstein

Medications and Supplements

If you are overseeing a person on prescription medicine, retest blood levels every 6-12 months. Good examples are thyroid meds and progesterone. This also applies to supplements that require blood work to monitor levels—vitamin D, DHEA, homocysteine, etc.

Remember this rule of thumb: The only thing that stays the same is change. A patient's needs will change over time as their body gets healthier. They will feel better a year after they started. They will feel much better two years later than a year ago. They will feel better at five years than at two years. And their medication(s) doses and supplement needs will probably change as well.

Lab Tests

Blood work should be done at least yearly for the reasons outlined above. When it comes to saliva and stool testing, once a person feels well and the repeat labs improve enough, you don't need to retest. Only retest if there is a significant new issue, or if the old issues return.

Consider a couple of examples. Retest saliva cortisol if a person has had new emotional trauma, once again isn't sleeping, or the anxiety/worry level that had dropped from an 8/10 to a 2-3/10 is now a 7/10. Or, with the stool test, all GI issues (and multiorgan system dysfunction in general because the gut is an important central mechanism) that had cleared are returning after another practitioner gave them an antibiotic for a sinus infection, or they got traveler's diarrhea while out of the country. They need to be retested.

Note: Treat the patient; not the lab tests. If a patient feels 80-100% better, but their lab results look so-so, it's okay to stop fixing what you're seeing on the lab results. Let them go, at least for the time being. It is the patient's quality of life that is most important. If they are living a happy and fulfilled life, "The Autoimmune Lifestyle," your work was done well. Reassess them during the annual consultation, or earlier if backsliding in symptom control begins.

On the other hand, if a patient still feels bad despite the interventions, methodically work through all the findings on testing and keep retesting at the appropriate intervals until they feel 70-100% better.

PROVIDING SUPPLEMENT ACCESS TO YOUR PATIENTS

Go confidently in the direction of your dreams! Live the life you've imagined.

—Henry David Thoreau

Why is it vital to encourage patients not to use the products they find at their local chain stores? The quality of supplements found over-the-counter are almost always poor. Unfortunately, the supplement industry is not held to the same standards of purity and content as the pharmaceutical industry.

By law, pharmaceutical companies must guarantee the purity and content of their products. Purity means the product has nothing in it that it shouldn't. The content means that the product contains what is listed on the label. They ensure this by having outside lab companies test their products to confirm purity and content before consumers use the products. In reality, the pharmaceutical industry uses many ingredients as fillers that patients with autoimmunity issues should not consume. Even gluten gets added! Or cornstarch, lactose, artificial dyes, etc.

In the supplement industry, no such requirements for purity and content are required prior to the sale of the products to the consumer. When you pick up a bottle from the shelf of a local chain store and examine the ingredients, you have no idea what is inside. A New York state study from a few years ago looked at the purity and content of hundreds of supplement products found in various stores. The authors' conclusion was that, in effect, most of the stuff was nothing more than ground-up house plants. The attorney general of the state of New York was so appalled that he temporarily pulled all over-the-counter supplements off all the shelves in every store in the entire state. One of the stores selling the poor quality supplements said in a statement that they "had no idea this was the case."[100] Yeah, right. The stores claim this while selling a thousand capsules of something for $20. They are not high-quality products when you can get a thousand capsules for $20.

Conflicting information can also lead to confusion in practitioners and patients alike. One study in a prominent medical journal may say that everyone should be on a multivitamin given how vitamin and mineral deficiencies are such huge drivers of chronic disease and our food supply is devoid of nutrient content these days. While at the same time another study, done as a longitudinal study in a stable community over three decades, may find no better outcomes in the individuals who took a multivitamin regularly over all those years compared to those who did not.

How can we reconcile this seemingly contradictory scientific data? Easy! We can recognize the poor quality of over-the-counter supplements. Knowing they don't contain what it says on the label and any high-quality ingredients used are in such low quantities (to sell 1,000 capsules for $20), it's easy to see that people who take these supplements are never getting a significant benefit. It makes perfect sense they were no healthier than the people who did not take the poor quality vitamins. It would be a total shock if the folks who took those over-the-counter vitamins for those 30 years were any healthier. Thus, it is not "conflicting scientific data," after all. Knowing the state of the typical supplement industry and federal regulations (or lack thereof), all this data is consistent with the known science.

We need to help our patients find "nutraceuticals" rather than supplements. Nutraceuticals are from specific companies that choose to have their products tested by outside firms for purity and content. Just as the pharmaceutical industry is required to do by the FDA, these nutraceutical companies abide by the same strict regulations.

To help your patients reverse and prevent all autoimmunity (and chronic disease in general), help them understand the difference between over-the-counter supplements and nutraceuticals. And, help them find the correct nutraceuticals so they can feel their best over time.

WHY PROVIDE SPECIFIC SUPPLEMENTS THROUGH YOUR OFFICE

Having an easy-to-access supply of nutraceuticals can be essential. Reversing and preventing chronic disease is not easy for patients. Not as easy as saying, "fill this prescription at your pharmacy and take one pill a day."

This approach won't work—it is putting a band-aid on a deeper problem and lets chronic disease create new issues over time. You want to make lifestyle changes, including taking the best nutraceuticals, as easy for each patient as possible. Having these nutraceuticals in your office can <u>dramatically</u> increase the chances the patient will follow your recommendations. On the other hand, it requires a significant financial investment to stock a closet (which should have a lock for safety) full of even the minimum number of products to reverse all autoimmunity. Further, these funds invested will be unavailable until these products are sold. That can tie up a lot of cash flow. Also, some practitioners are uncomfortable with the thought of benefiting financially from their patients' nutraceutical needs. Remember, you are providing a tremendous service to your patients when it comes to reversing their chronic diseases and preventing new ones. This is a service that many other practitioners cannot provide. Also, you will spend more time with them one-on-one during office visits than other practitioners would spend. A level 4 office visit can be billed by simply ordering a prescription medication due to the inherent risk of side effects and the need to monitor this toxic medication. Even if the practitioner spent two minutes with the patient. You, on the other hand, will want to bill based on time with autoimmunity patients. Therefore, you will need to spend 30-39 minutes on a patient's case during a follow-up visit to bill that same level 4 visit code. Or, 40-54 minutes for a level 5 visit. Or, 69 minutes for a level 5 visit plus the new prolonged services code 99417 (for more details on the new 2021 E/M office code guidelines, please go to *www.DrDavidBilstrom. com/npadguide*). The potential financial benefit from providing high-quality nutraceuticals to patients through your office can offset the potential loss of revenue (if you are someone who, until now, would spend six minutes with a patient and often use medications that would justify a level 4 visit) that might come from spending more time with each patient. It should be noted, however, the new 2021 E/M office code guidelines allow practitioners to bill for the entire time spent on a patient's case; not just face-to-face! Thus, going over lab results before entering the exam room is now billable time!

Think of it this way: providing these high-quality nutraceuticals to patients through your office will allow you to spend valuable time with them. It is the time they need to get the best possible care when it comes to reversing and preventing all chronic diseases.

If you are not ready to provide nutraceuticals through your office, either because of financial limitations or the thought of benefiting financially is uncomfortable, there are other options available.

SUPPLEMENTS THROUGH WWW.DRDAVIDBILSTROM.COM/STORE

One option for getting nutraceuticals that have been independently tested for purity and content is by having your patients visit my online store at *www.DrDavidBilstrom.com/store*. As time goes by, you may choose to have nutraceuticals available in your own office or website for the reasons discussed above. As you become more familiar with nutraceuticals and how they work in your distinctive patient population, modifying the products used most tends to occur. You may realize that you hardly ever use a product you thought would be important. If you had stocked your own office with it, the unused bottles would expire and now they cannot be sold. Over the years, hundreds of bottles have expired in my offices. It doesn't happen as often now as it did when I first started years ago. I also have simplified the number of products needed to do the work. At first, after all my advanced training in this type of medicine, I stocked my office with way too many unnecessary supplements. I only needed a core set of products that get used all the time. The exotic products for unique circumstances never got used because the patient's body healed on its own as we addressed the "biggest fish to fry." We didn't need the exotic products, after all. This store, on the other hand, already has the most effective and most popular products I have used over the years. It will also allow the patients to go to only one online store to procure all the best nutraceuticals, from the various companies discussed in this book.

Rather than having to go to multiple stores to get products from multiple manufacturers on their own, remember this: The process of making the appropriate changes needs to be as simple as possible to have the best chance for the patient to find the relief they are looking for.

For a list of supplements mentioned in this book, in alphabetical order and by company, with typical doses visit *www.DrDavidBilstrom.com/ npadguide.*

COMPOUNDED MEDICATIONS

The use of compounded medications (and even compounded nutraceuticals at times) will make available to your patients' products that are not normally available. For example, the compounded BiEst (c-BiEst) form is not available as a liquid version as opposed to a non-bioidentical pill or capsule form. Further, compounding a product in a cleaner form than is dispensed by prescription may be considered. For instance, "filler-free and dye-free" versions of medicines are routinely not available, such as Progesterone. Some patients are so sensitive, they can only tolerate the compounding pharmacy's versions with no dyes or fillers.

Finding the appropriate compounding pharmacy is crucial. Not only one that has the expertise but also one that can answer your questions as well as guide you with specific patient situations. My favorite is Pharmacy Solutions in Ann Arbor, Michigan. Not only can they do all of the above, but they ship to almost every state in the US. Their lead Ph.D. pharmacologist, Sahar Swidan, is one of the smartest people I have ever met. She has lectured all over the world for decades, regarding the reversal and prevention of chronic disease. She can be a great resource. I highly recommend you get to know her over time. For her contact information go to *www.DrDavidBilstrom. com/npadguide.*

TESTING KITS

Keep a few of each type of testing kit in your office. Set up an account with each company and they will send the kits. They are free of charge and last for a long time. The patient co-pays the testing company, if necessary, the company bills the rest to insurance. Complete the requisition, sign the form, and give the patient the kit to go home with. Each company can walk you through the process. Another option is to have the kits sent from the testing companies to the patients.

One exception to this is the food sensitivity test (FST.) This one is never covered by insurance and the patient will need to pay your office for the kit. The company will then bill your office the base kit fee. This test is a capillary finger prick test. The patient can take the kit home and do it themselves (or for their children) and then mail it in. Or your staff can administer the test, let the blood spots dry, and then take it to the post office that day. To cover the time required by your staff to do the FST activities, charge the patient more than the base cost.

Doctor's Data, Inc. Comprehensive Stool Analysis (Digestive stool analysis), Urine Toxic Metals (Heavy metal test)
3755 Illinois Avenue
St. Charles, IL 60174-2420
USA
US and Canada 800.323.2784
UK 0871.218.0052
Global +1.630.377.8139
Global Fax +1.630.587.7860
Email: *info@doctorsdata.com*
doctorsdata.com

Genova Diagnostics. GI Effects Profile (Digestive stool analysis), Stress Profile Cortisol (Saliva Cortisol and DHEA), and One Day Hormone Check (Saliva hormones including sex hormones, cortisol/ DHEA, and Melatonin)
63 Zillicoa Street

Asheville, North Carolina 28801
USA
US 800.522.4762
Global +1.800.522.4762
Email: *info@gdx.net*
Gdx.net

US BioTek Laboratories. 96 General Food Panel (Food sensitivity test)
16020 Linden Ave N.
Shoreline, WA 98133
USA
USA and Canada Toll-Free +1.877.318.8728
+1.206.365.1256
Fax: +1.206.363.8790
cservice@usbiotek.com
usbiotek.com

ADDENDUM

The future belongs to those who believe in the beauty of their dreams.

—ELEANOR ROOSEVELT

Look for the companion book for NPs, but also the public at large, to be published next. This will provide more detailed information on many of the subjects presented here. For example, more details on thyroid restoration and cortisol, the forgotten hormone.

By necessity, in this "Nurse Practitioners' Guide to Autoimmune Medicine," we are focused on brevity. A guide that could be read as a book and a quick reference for patient treatment. But also, a guide to building your practice in autoimmune medicine and become the local "expert" on the subject.

The future book will provide more information on why our work to change the way we treat autoimmune disease is critical. That, along with this "Guide", will put you in a position not only to continue the revolution of the Nurse Practitioner as an independent medical practitioner but to become the expert in your community on the reversal and prevention of all autoimmune disease. At least 50 million Americans need help with the reversal of their current autoimmune disease, as well as countless untold accounts of people who need help with preventing them in the first place. Be their guide to better health when the rest of the world tells them there's nothing else that can be done.

DEDICATION

The author would like to lift the goblet of vintage computer text to his fabulous content editor Katie Rose Waechter, line editor E.M. Kinga Mac, and the dynamic sister duo "changing the way autoimmune disease is treated worldwide", Jessica Allen and Ginger Allen. This book would never have happened without their compassion, knowledge, dedication, and beautiful souls. My wife Jody for her unwavering support and love over these many years both in the clinic and at home. My parents for being the parents I needed to find my way to medicine and for having instilled in me the importance of a life spent helping others. To Tom Robbins, for reigniting a love of books and giving me the idea that having lived an eclectic life, including spending a chunk of time in Thailand, may be just what is necessary for becoming a writer. And for Switters. And to the Artist's Cafe, forever across the street from the Art Institute of Chicago in my mind, for always helping me remember my beloved grandmother, Elizabeth, and for a favor given me years ago at a time when it was so needed.

REFERENCES

1. Autoimmune Disease Statistics. (n.d.). AARDA. *https://www. aarda.org/news-information/statistics/.*

2. Wren. (2016, February 6). Weighing the risks: Glenn frey and RD drugs. RheumatoidArthritis.Net. *https://rheumatoidarthritis.net/ living/weighing-the-risks-glenn-frey-and-drugs/*

3. Araújo-Fernandez S. et al. Drug-induced Lupus: Including anti-tumour necrosis factor and interferon induced. Lupus 2014: 23(6): 545-553.

4. Caspi R. (2008). Immunotherapy of autoimmunity and cancer: the penalty for success. Nat Rev Immunol, 8(12), 970–976.

5. Boelaert K. et al. (2010). Prevalence and relative risk of other autoimmune diseases in subjects with autoimmune thyroid disease. Am J Med, 123(2), 183.e1–183.e9.

6. Anaya J.-m. et al. (2016). The autoimmune ecology. Front Immunol, 7(139).

7. Kivity S. et al. (2011). Vitamin D and autoimmune thyroid diseases. Cell Mol Immunol, 8(3), 243–247.

8. Delitala A.P. et al. (2017). Thyroid hormones, metabolic syndrome and its components. Endocr Metab Immune Disord Drug Targets, 17(1), 56–62.

9. Joseph J. et al. (2015). Diurnal salivary cortisol, glycemia and insulin resistance: The multi-ethnic study of atherosclerosis. Psychoneuroendocrinology, 62, 327–335.

10. Worthington J. (2015). The intestinal immunoendocrine axis: novel cross-talk between enteroendocrine cells and the immune

system during infection and inflammatory disease. Biochem Soc Trans, 43(4), 727–733.

11. Kabouridis P.S., Pachnis V. (2015). Emerging roles of gut microbiota and the immune system in the development of the enteric nervous system. J Clin Invest, 125(3), 956–964.

12. Chen C.Q. et al. (2011). Distribution, function and physiological role of melatonin in the lower gut. World J Gastroenterol, 17(34), 3888–3898.

13. Accurate education-melatonin. (n.d.). Accurate Clinic. *http://accurateclinic.com/accurate-education-melatonin/*.

14. Furness J.B. et al. (1999). Nutrient testing and signaling mechanisms in the gut. The intestine as a sensory organ: neural, endocrine, and immune responses. Am J Physiol, 277(5), 6922–6928.

15. Castro-Nallar E. et al. (2015). Composition, taxonomy and functional diversity of the oropharynx microbiome in individuals with schizophrenia and controls. PeerJ, 3, e1140.

16. Schenkein H.A., Loos B.G. (2015). Inflammatory mechanisms linking periodontal disease to cardiovascular disease. J Clin Periodontol, 40(Suppl 14), 51–s69.

17. Hoggard M. et al. (2017). Chronic rhinosinusitis and the evolving understanding of microbial ecology in chronic inflammatory mucosal disease. Clin Microbiol Rev, 30(1), 321–348.

18. What is celiac disease? (n.d.). Celiac Disease Foundation. *https://celiac.org/about-celiac-disease/what-is-celiac-disease/*

19. Symptoms of Celiac Disease. (n.d.). Celiac Disease Foundation. *https://celiac.org/about-celiac-disease/symptoms-of-celiac-disease/*

20. Home—Coeliac Australia. (2020). Coeliac Australia. *https://www.coeliac.org.au/*

21. Johnson J. et al. (1836). The medico-chirurgical review and journal of practical medicine (vol. 24). Richard George S Wood.

22. Sakihara S. et al. (2010). Evaluation of plasma, salivary, and urinary cortisol levels for diagnosis of Cushing's syndrome. Endocr J, 57(4), 331–337.

23. Tsigos C., Chrousos G.P. (2002). Hypothalamic-pituitary-adrenal axis, neuroendocrine factors and stress. J Psychosom Res, 53(4), 865–871.

24. de J R De-Paula V et al. (2018). Relevance of gut microbiota in cognition, behavior and Alzheimer's disease. Pharmacol Res, 136, 29–34.

25. Kieffer DA. et al. (2016). Impact of dietary fibers on nutrient management and detoxification organs: Gut, liver and kidneys. Adv Nutr, 7(6), 1111–1121.

26. Patel S. et al. (2018). Estrogen: The necessary evil for human health, and ways to tame it. Biomed Pharmacother, 102, 403–411.

27. Vojdani A. et al. (2014). Environmental triggers and autoimmunity. Autoimmune Dis 2014, 798029.

28. Estimates of prevalence for autoimmune disease. (2020, November 18). The Autoimmune Registry. *https://www.autoimmuneregistry.org/autoimmune-statistics*

29. Fairweather D., Rose N.R. (2004). Women and autoimmune diseases. Emerg Infect Dis, 10(11), 2005–2011.

30. Machi S. et al. (2004). The national burdens of rheumatoid arthritis and osteoarthritis in Japan: Projections to the year 2010, with future changes in severity distribution. Mod Rheum, 14(4), 285–290.

31. Yamanaka H. et al. (2014). Estimates of the prevalence of and current treatment practices for rheumatoid arthritis in Japan using reimbursement data from health insurance societies and IORRA cohort. Mod Rheumatol, 24(1), 33–40.

32. Swidan, S., Bennett, M. (2021) Advanced Therapeutics in Pain Medicine. CRC Press.

33. Chang C.Y. et al. (2009). Essential fatty acids and human brain. Acta Neurol Taiwan, 18(4), 231–241.

34. Lanphear B. et al. (2018). Low-level lead exposure and mortality in US adults: A population-based cohort study. Lancet, 3(4), e177–e184.

35. Nawrot T., Staessen J.A. (2006). Low-level environmental exposure to lead unmasked as silent killer. Circulation, 114(13), 1347–1349.

36. Lead (Pb) Toxicity: What is the Biological Fate of Lead in the Body? | ATSDR—Environmental Medicine & Environmental Health Education—CSEM. (2019, June 12). Agency for Toxic Substances and Disease Registry. *https://www.atsdr.cdc.gov/csem/csem.asp?csem=34&po=9*

37. Pizzorno J. (2015). Is challenge testing valid for assessing body metal burden? Integ Med, 14(4), 8–14.

38. Crinnion W.J. (2009). The benefits of pre-and post-challenge urine heavy metal testing: Part 1. Altern Med Rev, 14(1), 3–8.

39. Crinnion W.J. (2009). The benefit of pre- and post-challenge urine heavy metal testing: Part 2. Altern Med Rev, 14(2), 103–108.

40. Kubasik N.P., Volosin M.T. (1973). Heavy metal poisoning: clinical aspects and laboratory analysis. Am J MedTechnol, 39(11), 443–450.

41. Efstratiadis G. et al. (2006). Hypomagnesemia and cardiovascular system. Hippokratia, 10(4), 147–152.

42. Ali A. et al. (2017). Efficacy of individualized diets in patients with irritable bowel syndrome: A randomized controlled trial. BMJ Open Gastroenterol, 4(1), e000164.

43. Gupta M. et al. Diagnosis of food allergy. Immunol Allergy Clin North Am 2018; 38(1): 39-52.

44. Gordon B. R. Approaches to testing for food and chemical sensitivities. Otolaryngol Clin North Am 2003; 36(5): 917-940.

45. Wahls T. (2014). The Wahls Protocol. Penguin Group.

46. Brown N., Panksepp J. (2009). Low-dose naltrexone for disease prevention and quality of life. Med Hypotheses, 72(3), 333–337.

47. Munger K. et al. (2016). Vitamin D status during pregnancy and risk of multiple sclerosis in offspring of women in the Finnish maternity cohort. JAMA Neurol, 73(5), 515–519.

48. Hypponeu E. et al. (2001). Intake of vitamin D and type 1 diabetes: A birth-cohort study. Lancet, 358(9292), 1500–1503.

49. McDonnell S. et al. (2018). Breast cancer-risk markedly lower with serum 25-hydroxy vitamin D concentrations > 60 vs <20 ng/ml (150 vs 50 nmol/L): Pooled analysis of two randomized trials and a prospective cohort. PLOS. doi:10.1371/journal.pone.0199265

50. Garland C. et al. (2006). The role of vitamin D in cancer prevention. Am J Public Health, 96(2), 252–261.

51. Bakke D., Sun J. (2018). Ancient nuclear receptor VDR with new functions: microbiome and inflammation. Inflamm Bowel Dis, 24(6), 1149–1154.

52. Ginde A. et al. (2009). Demographic differences and trends in vitamin D insufficiency in the US population, 1988–2004. Arch Intern Med, 169(6), 626–632.

53. Gupta P.G. (2014). Role of iron (Fe) in body. IOSR JAC, 7(11).

54. Boldyrev A. et al. (2013). Why is homocysteine toxic for the nervous and immune systems?. Curr Aging Sci, 6(1), 29–36.

55. Perla-Kajan J. et al. (2007). Mechanisms of homocysteine toxicity in humans. Amino Acids, 32(4), 561–572.

56. Egnell M. et al.(2017). B-vitamin intake from diet and supplements and breast cancer risk in women: Results from the prospective NutriNet-Sante cohort. Nutrients, 9(5).

57. Dai Z., Koh W.P. (2015). B-vitamins and bone health-a review of the current evidence. Nutrients, 7(5), 3322–3346.

58. Kaluzna-Czaplinska J. (2013). A focus on homocysteine in autism. Acta Biochim Pol, 60(2), 137–142.

59. Altun H. et al. (2018). The levels of vitamin D, vitamin D receptors, homocysteine and complex B vitamin in children with autism spectrum disorders. Clin Psychopharmacol Neurosci, 16(4), 383–390.

60. Oikonomidi A. et al. (2016). Homocysteine metabolism is associated with cerebrospinal fluid levels of soluble amyloid precursor protein and amyloid beta. J Neurochem, 139(2), 324–332.

61. McCully K.S. (2017). Hyperhomocysteinemia, suppressed immunity, and altered oxidative metabolism caused by pathologic microbes in atherosclerosis and dementia. Front Aging Neurosci, 9, 324.

62. McCully K.S. (2016). Homocysteine, infections, polyamines, oxidative metabolism, and the pathogenesis of dementia and atherosclerosis. J Alzheimers Dis, 54(4), 1283–1290.

63. Patterson S. et al. (2007). Major metabolic homocysteine-derivative, homocysteine thiolactone, exerts changes in pancreatic beta-cell glucose sensing, cellular signal transduction and integrity. Arch Biochem Biophys, 461(2), 287–293.

64. Gominak S.C. (2016). Vitamin D deficiency changes the intestinal microbiota reducing B vitamin production in the gut. The resulting lack of Pantothenic Acid adversely affects the immune system, producing a 'pro-inflammatory' state associated with atherosclerosis and autoimmunity. Med Hypotheses, 94, 103–107.

65. Shandal V., Luo J.J. (2016). Clinical manifestations of isolated elevated homocysteine-induced peripheral neuropathy in adults. J Clin Neuromuscul Dis, 17(3), 106–109.

66. Solomon L.R. (2016). Vitamin B-12 responsive neuropathies: A case series. Nutr Neurosci, 19(4), 162–168.

67. Solomon L.R. (2016). Functional vitamin B-12 deficiency in advanced malignancy: Implications for the management of neuropathy and neuropathic pain. Support Care Cancer, 24(8), 3489–3494.

68. Santos K.F. et al. (2005). The prima donna of epigenetics: The regulation of gene expression by DNA methylation. Braz J Med Biol Res, 38(10), 1531–1541.

69. Peterson S.J. et al. (2016). Is a normal TSH synonymous with 'Euthyroidism' in levothyroxine monotherapy? J Clin Endocrinol Metab, 101(12), 4964–4973.

70. Statistics. (2016, May 10). About IBS: International Foundation for Gastrointestinal Disorders. *https://www.aboutibs.org/facts-about-ibs/statistics.html*

71. Body burden: The pollution in newborns. (2005, July 14). Environmental Working Group. *https://www.ewg.org/research/body-burden-pollution-newborns*

72. Tivesten Å et al. (2014). Dehydroepiandrosterone and its sulfate predict the 5-year risk of coronary heart disease events in elderly men. J Am Coll Cardiol, 64(17), 1801–1810.

73. Jimenez M. et al. (2013). Low dehydroepiandrosterone sulphate is associated with increased risk of ischemic stroke among women. Stroke, 44(7), 1784–1789.

74. Pluchino N. et al. (2015). Neurobiology of DHEA and effects on sexuality, mood and cognition. J Steroid Biochem Mol Biol, 145, 273–280.

75. Ernster L., Dallner G. (1995). Biochemical, physiological and medical aspects of ubiquinone function. Biochim Biophys Acta, 1271(1), 195–204.

76. Nielsen T.R. et al. (2007). Multiple sclerosis after infectious mononucleosis. Arch Neurol, 64(1), 72–75.

77. Handel A.E. et al. (2010). An updated meta-analysis of the risk of multiple sclerosis following infectious mononucleosis. PLOS ONE, 5(9).

78. Silver as a drinking-water disinfectant. (2018). World Health Organization. *https://www.who.int/water_sanitation_health/publications/silver-02032018.pdf?ua=1*

79. Railean-Plugaru V. et al. (2016). Antimicrobial properties of biosynthesized silver nanoparticles studied by flow cytometry and related techniques. Electrophoresis, 37(5–6), 752–761.

80. Khan S. et al. (2018). Nanosilver: New ageless and versatile biomedical therapeutic scaffold. Int J Nanomed, 13, 733–762.

81. Kelly D. M., Jones T. H. Testosterone: a metabolic hormone in health and disease. J Endocrinol 2013; 217(3): R25-R45.

82. Kaltenboeck, A. et al. (2012). US privately insured employees with hypogonadism. J Sex Med 2012; 9(9): 2438-2447.

83. Murkes D. et al. Percutaneous estradiol/oral micronized progesterone has less adverse effects and different gene regulation than oral conjugated equine estrogens/medroxyprogesterone acetate in the breasts of healthy women in vivo. Gynecol Endocrinol 2012; 28(Suppl 2): 21-25.

84. Goodman M. P. Are all estrogens created equal? A review of oral vs transdermal therapy. J Womens Health (Larchmt) 2012; 21(2): 161-169.

85. Mendelsohn M., Karas R.H. (1999). The protective effects of estrogen on the cardiovascular system. N Engl J Med, 340(23), 1801–1811.

86. O'Leary P. et al. (2000). Salivary, but not serum or urinary levels of progesterone are elevated after topical application of progesterone cream to pre and postmenopausal women. Clin Endocrinol, 53(5), 615–620.

87. Hughes G.C., Choubey D. (2014). Modulation of autoimmune rheumatic diseases by oestrogen and progesterone. Nat Rev Rheumatol, 10(12), 740–751.

88. Westaby D. et al. (1977). Liver damage from long-term methyl-testosterone. Lancet, 2(8032), 262–263.

89. Selye H. (1950). Stress and the general adaptation syndrome. Br Med J, 1(4667), 1383–1392.

90. McEwen B. (2008). Protecting and damaging effects of stress mediators. N Engl J Med, 338, 171–179.

91. Kumar P. et al. (2008). Exocrine dysfunction correlates with endocrinal impairment of pancreas in type 2 diabetes mellitus. Indian J Endocrinol Metab, 22(1), 121–125.

92. Menees S.B. et al. (2015). A meta-analysis of the utility of C-reactive protein, erythrocyte sedimentation rate, fecal calprotectin, and fecal lactoferrin to exclude inflammatory bowel disease in adults with IBS. Am J Gastroenterol, 110(3), 444–454.

93. Dabritz J. et al. (2014). Diagnostic utility of faecal biomarkers in patients with irritable bowel syndrome. World J Gastroenterol, 20(2), 363–375.

94. Parsons K. et al. (2014). Novel testing enhances irritable bowel syndrome medical management: The IMMINENT study. Glob Acv. Health Med, 3(3), 25–32.

95. Masters S.B. et al. (2019). Katzurg and Trevor's pharmacology: Examination and board review, 18th ed. McGraw Hill Medical, 481–483.

96. Magnesium in diet. (2020, November 3). MedlinePlus. *https://medlineplus.gov/ency/article/002423.htm*

97. Tengrup I. et al. (1981). Influence on zinc synthesis and the accumulation of collagen in early granulation tissue. Surg Gynecol Obstet, 152(3), 323–326.

98. Celiac disease—Diagnosis and treatment—Mayo Clinic. (2020, October 21). Mayo Clinic. *https://www.mayoclinic.org/diseases-conditions/celiac-disease/diagnosis-treatment/drc-20352225*

99. Chandrasekhar K. et al. (2012). A prospective, randomized double-blind, placebo controlled study of safety and efficacy of a high-concentration full-spectrum extract of Ashwagandha root in reducing stress and anxiety in adults. Indian J Psychol Med, 34(3), 255–262.

100. New York Attorney General Targets Supplements at Major Retailers. (2015, February 3). The New York Times. *https://well. blogs.nytimes.com/2015/02/03/new-york-attorney-general-targets-supplements-at-major-retailers/*

Printed in the USA
CPSIA information can be obtained
at www.ICGtesting.com
LVHW011042030923
757096LV00005B/13